THE F

Tish Hayton was born in Christchurch, Hampshire and educated at Oxford and Leicester Universities. She now lives in St Albans with her husband and two teenage sons.

By the age of fourteen, Tish had a weight problem which lasted for the next twenty-eight years. When in 1984 her youngest son was diagnosed as being intolerant to four particular foods she was incredulous, but decided to give the treatment a chance before dismissing the idea. The results were so encouraging that she decided to try out a similar diet on herself: within days, her energy had increased enormously and her permanent hunger had disappeared. Over the next few weeks she lost a stone in weight and she saw a great improvement in her health. She then enlisted 100 volunteers via a plea on local radio to find out if it worked for them – in almost every case it did. This new way of eating forms the basis of THE FOOD ADDICT'S DIET.

The Food Addict's Diet

Tish Hayton

HEADLINE

To Dawn and Philip,
who started it all,
and to Anne,
who believed in me

First published in 1991
by HEADLINE BOOK PUBLISHING PLC

10 9 8 7 6 5 4 3 2

ISBN 0 7472 3476 0

Typeset in 10/11 pt Times
by Colset Private Limited, Singapore

Printed and bound by
Collins Manufacturing, Glasgow

HEADLINE BOOK PUBLISHING PLC
Headline House,
79 Great Titchfield Street
London W1P 7FN

Contents

Acknowledgements

I would like to thank through these pages everyone who took part in the diet trials during 1988 and 1989. Thank you also to BBC Radio Bedfordshire, the *St Albans Review* and the *Harpenden Herald* for the coverage they gave me. Thank you to Murray, Lynn, Hazel and Sylvia, who spent hours looking over the manuscript. I am greatly indebted to Beebug of St Albans for a continuous supply of paper and other computer equipment, and to the various daytime presenters of BBC Radio 1 who kept me sane throughout. Many, many thanks to Sally Holloway for her patience and stoicism in making sense of the manuscript and, above all, thanks to my family, who patiently put up with it all.

Note
If you are pregnant or are taking any form of medication, consult a doctor before undertaking any new diet.

Introduction

This is a diet to bring back the joy of eating. It is the diet for today, because in the rush of our everyday lives we seem to have forgotten that food can bring us pleasure and health in one delicious package. Food should be at the centre of our lives, not pushed like a guilty secret into a corner out of the way. So if you find food a problem in any way, this is the diet for you.

You are probably reading this book because you want to lose weight. Well, with the Food Addict's Diet you can – easily, gently and effectively – but this is much, much more than just a slimming diet. The advice in this book will be your gateway to a totally new eating experience and a new idea: food addiction.

Food addiction is responsible for most of the problems we have with food today. Food addiction creates an addictive craving which is often mistaken for greed, and can have profound but subtle effects on your eating habits. It works on a sliding scale: it can be as slight as a subtle inclination that you hardly notice towards a few favourite foods, or as powerful as a compulsive desire to eat large quantities of particular 'binge' foods.

Addictive cravings can be revealed by your eating habits, and by noticing your cravings you will be able to see how much of an addict you are. An addiction to a food drives you to eat at least a little of it every day of your life, so any food that you eat daily could be a sign of a growing dependency.

1

WHY SLIMMING DIETS DON'T WORK

If you are a food addict, like addicts of all kinds, you probably find it hard to do without the food you are addicted to for very long. If you are overweight, and must cut down the amount you eat, or cut out some foods altogether, you will lapse again and again, drawn back to your favourite foods by your cravings for them. I believe that food addiction is the main reason why slimming diets are so hard to follow and why they so often break down.

The Food Addict's Diet will do more than just cut down your food consumption to help you lose weight. It will address the real problem behind the weight: your lack of control over your eating habits.

Why do all slimmers stick to a diet for a while and lose weight but then return to their old habits and gain it again? Why do they torture themselves, struggling to deny their natural instincts to eat, and constantly inventing new methods to keep their food consumption down? Anyone can lose weight. Losing weight is possible for anyone on any slimming diet, provided you stick with it for long enough.

Slimming diets are usually boring. They make you feel deprived, they are antisocial, and they isolate you from other people. Above all, they are very, very hard to stick to in the early stages. I would guess that 90 per cent of slimming diets fail in the first three days. This book will explain exactly why we all feel so deprived and unhappy at the beginning of a new diet, and also why we so often fail.

This is the first diet where you will be *encouraged* to break it at least once! You will be invited to have a 'diet rest' at an appointed time, and then you will see clearly the effect of that diet lapse on your appetite. With the help of this exercise you will realise why you have never stayed with a slimming diet before: you do not lack will power, neither are you a freak. You are a food addict, and before you can follow a slimming diet you must learn to cope with your addiction to those high-calorie foods. You can do this with the help of the Food Addict's Diet.

Once your addictions and your appetite are firmly under your control, you will be able to keep to a healthy slimming regime and see good results. Not only that, but the Food Addict's Diet will give you something no other diet can offer: when your good intentions begin to fade, you will not give up in despair at your own weakness. You will at last understand why you failed, and know how to begin again. This is how you will succeed: by learning how to cope with your failures!

OVERWEIGHT AND FOOD INTOLERANCE

I began researching into the effects of food on health in 1984, and I quickly discovered an interesting link between food intolerance and excess weight. People who are intolerant of certain foods tend to become 'addicted' to the very foods that cause them to react. This means that if you show signs of food addiction, you may also be intolerant to the very foods you crave.

Some symptoms of food intolerance can greatly aggravate the problem of excess weight by adding extra inches. This particularly applies to people who suffer fluid retention or abdominal bloating, both of which are recognised signs of food intolerance. People who suffer from fluid retention feel swollen all over. People who suffer from abdominal bloating carry most of their weight around their waist and their stomach tends to protrude.

Persistent minor symptoms, such as headaches, aching limbs or a lack of energy, are often put down to 'nerves' or 'stress', but they can be caused by a physical reaction to some of the foods you eat every day. This diet is a useful way of finding out whether or not those symptoms you thought you would have to learn to live with are caused by food intolerance. Following this diet will also put an end to them.

THE THEORY BEHIND THE DIET

By 1987 I decided that if it was true that being overweight and food intolerance were closely linked, then a diet designed to cure food intolerance would also help people to lose weight.

My theory was that if you were intolerant to a high-calorie food such as cream, milk or cheese, and became addicted to it, you would eat too much of it and gain weight. You would also find it hard to reduce your consumption of it to follow a slimming diet.

Therefore to lose weight you would need to cure your addiction to the food. The only way to do this would be to remove it from your diet. This would also cure the symptoms of food intolerance and at the same time reduce your calorie intake. I set out to create just such a diet and see if this theory was true.

THE FOOD ADDICT'S DIET IS BORN

First of all, I tried out the theory on myself. I eliminated just four basic food ingredients from my diet while eating *as much as I liked* of all other foods. To my amazement, within a few weeks not only was I slimmer, but I was healthier, stronger, and felt more alive than I had done for ages. The way I now ate was healthy and satisfying, and I decided to stick with it.

A few weeks later, for various reasons, I ate the banned foods again, and was surprised at the bad effect this had on my arthritis and my swollen ankles. Despite the fact that my symptoms had at once become worse, I found it unexpectedly hard to make a start on the diet again. I soon realised that I was experiencing the effects of an addiction, rather than a lack of will power. Incredibly, for the first time in twenty-five years of slimming I did not have to feel a failure: instead, I was an addict! I stayed calm, waited till the following Monday, and simply began again. Suddenly it was so easy!

That was five years ago. I now know that my body has a problem handling wheat products and caffeine drinks, both of which have definite physical effects upon me. As far as I can, I have removed them from my life, and even now I feel a huge sense of relief that I no longer have to torture myself with slimming diet failure. My addictions were always the reason for my problems, and I now have them firmly under control. I have lost weight and, though I am not thin, I feel 'just right' – and that is all that matters, after all!

Discovering food addiction transformed my whole attitude to myself, and enabled me to come to terms with my weight. I felt at once that this joy should be shared with as many people as possible, so I decided to find out if this kind of diet would work as well for other people as it had for me. In 1987–8 I advertised for 'guinea pigs' on local radio and in the local newspapers.

Over a hundred people applied to try out the diet as an 'experiment' and fill in various questionnaires and reports. The vast majority of those who followed it over the three-week period felt much more energetic on the diet. To most it was a gentle and effective way of losing weight, but many of them found relief from depression, headaches and other symptoms. Later, they were able to see how these problems had been created by reactions to particular foods.

For some of my guinea pigs, their almost constant craving for food was so overwhelming that it had led to compulsive eating. This varied among individuals from occasional bingeing to a sixteen-year history of bulimia (regular bingeing and vomiting). Food addiction is a useful new approach for compulsive eaters, because it shows them that cravings are not all in the mind. It was through discussing their overwhelming desire for food that I realised that food addiction was much more damaging and widespread than I had ever imagined, and that it was high time we had a diet specially designed for food addicts.

HOW DOES THE DIET WORK?

AN EXPERIMENT

To try the Food Addict's Diet you begin with the three-week 'four zero experiment'. All this involves is avoiding completely just *four* ingredients while eating as *much as you like* of everything else. There is no restriction on how much food you eat during the experiment, for the first step is to cure your food addictions.

The foods that are eliminated are wheat, milk, sugar and potatoes, and all foods made from them. These will be known as the 'zero' foods, and I will explain in detail on page 18 why they have been singled out from all the other foods we eat.

Anyone who suffers from food intolerance will recognise this kind of diet, for it requires not just cutting down, but a *complete elimination* of the selected ingredients for the entire three weeks of the experiment. After this, the selected ingredients are deliberately reintroduced into the diet during the 'rest test' in order to see the effects of eating them again.

THE MAGIC

When you begin the experiment be prepared for all kinds of changes: probably for the first time in your life you will be living completely without four staple foods that you have eaten in some form or other every day.

After an interval of about four days, during which all kinds of readjustments will occur, your body will give a sigh of relief, and you will begin to feel really wonderful:

alive, strong, and full of a wonderful sense of lightness and clarity. This is the 'magic' of the Food Addict's Diet, and once you have experienced it you will want to feel that magic every day. Believe me, with the help of the advice in this book, you can.

KNOWING MORE ABOUT YOU

Through the challenge of the four zero experiment, you will learn a great deal about how your food exerts an influence over your appetite. By the end of the three weeks you will know if you are a food addict, and what you can do about it if you are.

By now you will know how to keep your appetite under control; keep your diet varied and prevent food addictions creeping back into your life; and you will also know whether particular foods are affecting your health.

LOSING WEIGHT PERMANENTLY

Some people find they lose weight while on the experiment. You do not count calories, fat units or fibre, and you can eat as much as you feel you need, because you will be using your body's natural controls to limit your food intake.

For those who are anxious to lose weight a little faster, there are six ways of accelerating weight loss given in Chapter 9, all firmly based in the idea of avoiding the four zero foods – but with a few extra refinements.

A SAFE ELIMINATION DIET

If you have already been advised to eliminate either milk, wheat, potatoes or sugar from your diet because of an allergy, or if you suspect that you may be intolerant to any of them, this book can be a helpful guide to keeping the balances of your diet correct while you eliminate them all at once.

The British diet is so firmly based upon these foods

that they turn up in almost every dish. Sticking to a diet eliminating any or all of them for many years can be very hard, and this book can help to make it easier, with all kinds of suggestions, safeguards and recipes.

DO I NEED THIS BOOK?

Yes! By picking up this book you have shown that at least a small part of you identifies with the idea of food addiction. There are two main groups of people that this way of eating can help: the overweight, and those suffering from the effects of food intolerance. In many cases these two categories overlap, and most people can learn something from trying the three-week experiment – as you can see from these true stories of four people who were helped by the Food Addict's Diet.

Sheila: The inside story of being heavily overweight

Sheila is fat: *really* fat. At twenty stones she is twice her recommended weight. Sheila sleeps on a specially strengthened single bed which is nearer the floor than normal.

She described one particular day to me, on which she had to go to her doctor for a check-up on a urinary problem. The bed creaked terribly as she got out of it and walked slowly to the bathroom. The mirror showed her face to be puffy and pale, her mouth a sour crease in her face. She drank black coffee and sat alone in her kitchen, already tired, silently staring, her mind a blank. Later she hurried to the bus stop, her breathing laboured.

At the doctor's she climbed the steps, panting.

The doctor, as usual, began with The Weight. 'How are you doing losing weight?' she asked brightly.

In reply, Sheila – as usual – lied: 'Very slow, doctor . . . but I am trying.'

Getting on to the narrow bed for the examination was a nightmare. The nurse had to come in to give a hand.

8

Sheila made a joke about a block and tackle. In the midst of the laughter, she submitted her weary body to the examination, staring at the ceiling, red-faced with shame.

Afterwards, she rushed into work, panting, flustered and redder than ever. Sheila was a switchboard operator for a large chemical company. Sitting on her stool at the switchboard her Other Life took over. Her great gift is her voice: warm, mellow and filled with life.

When you speak to Sheila on the phone, you speak to the real Sheila, not the great body that she lives in. Her clientele like her jolly ways, but of course they never see her in the flesh. Seven years ago Sheila was a prize-winner at her slimming club as she lost four and a half stones. She is now heavier than she was before she began that particular diet and is too ashamed to go back.

Sheila's story is the story of every severely overweight person: locked into a distorted, unattractive body, angry, frustrated and despairing, the need to solve this problem is beginning to eclipse everything else in life. That 'big, jolly lady' you meet on the bus may be laughing, but deep inside she is unhappy and alone with a problem that she sees as 'her fault'.

Sheila's 'cure' began almost at once. As soon as we began to discuss why she was unable to stick to a diet, she began to feel better about herself. I told her that she was not weak-willed or greedy: she was simply addicted to food, and there was a way to bring that addiction under control.

Gradually, Sheila is learning how to feed her body the food it really needs. She has much more energy and is gradually and naturally losing weight. Above all, she now enjoys her food, and eats well without gaining weight. She is already slimmer than she has been for years, and confidently talks about the time when she will be able to buy 'proper' clothes again.

Wendy: Overweight and food intolerant

Wendy was three stones overweight and suffered from fluid retention, digestive disorders, insomnia, aching

9

limbs and attacks of breathlessness. She had been over-weight since babyhood, but she had never been able to shift it, even when sticking rigidly to very low-calorie diets. She was constantly tired, but drove herself very hard in her voluntary work. When I first met her she looked unhappy, swollen and exhausted.

Gradually, and with the help of weekly support consultations in the pilot 'Winners' Group (see page 301), Wendy changed her diet. She cut out the 'zero' foods, and introduced new ones, principally fish, nuts and seeds, into her diet. Her weekly eating reports gradually revealed more varied and increasingly healthy eating habits.

During the first week she didn't lose much weight, but she later admitted that she had 'cheated' once or twice for reasons she could not fully understand. I explained how insidious food addiction can be, and about the need to be watchful for unconscious 'excuses'. We decided that she should take great care to stick to the plan rigidly the next week.

A week later she was beginning to lose weight at last. She had slimmer ankles, more energy, and felt very happy and positive. With the change in diet came a feeling of inner peace. A nervous, churning feeling in her stomach that troubled her ceaselessly had stopped during that week.

The story still continues: sixty years of being overweight will not be overcome in a few months, but the experiment brought Wendy new hope and an increased sense of well-being. It is now quite clear that she has reactions to some of the food she eats. It seems that eating foods made with wheat flour increases her fluid retention, and aggravates the pains in her joints. Also, milk products and caffeine drinks give her headaches, and seem to affect her sleeping habits. Wendy now knows that for most of her life she has been made ill by her food, and one by one we are finding the suspects and removing them. As we do so, her health is slowly improving.

For sixty years Wendy's symptoms of food intolerance had remained unrecognised for what they were. Some of her symptoms – panic attacks and breathlessness – were very distressing and frightening, but medical tests showed nothing physically wrong. Eventually both Wendy and her doctor had begun to conclude that it was 'all in the mind'. How wrong they were!

Pamela: A 'binge/vomit' eater

Pamela was reluctant to tell me that, slim and bright as she was, she had an eating disorder. However, she soon discovered that I was not going to think her neurotic or crazy. To me, she was a food addict. I found her intelligent, sensitive and very rational. Until she told me about it, her bingeing and vomiting had been a closely guarded, shameful secret.

Pamela followed the diet very carefully for the first two weeks. Even after the first five days she told me with some surprise that she had not felt the need to vomit from the moment she had started the experiment. In fact, she actually managed to go for two weeks without vomiting: the longest she had managed since her problem began twelve years before. I then lost contact with her over the summer holidays, during which time her addiction dragged her back to her normal eating and vomiting pattern. However, she told me later that she had learned a lot about herself. She had never before thought of her cravings for food as an addiction, and never known that there was a practical way to avoid vomiting.

Some weeks later she decided to begin the plan again, but this time she was committed to follow it for as long as possible. She still attends regular psychotherapy sessions, but she has found her attitude changing, particularly her negative attitude to food itself. This eventually became clear to her psychotherapist. She has also changed the food she buys. She no longer goes shopping for 'binge food' such as white bread or chocolate. She now buys a wide variety of foods, and particularly fruit and vegetables. In her words, she has become a 'health nut' and is converting her husband to her new way of eating.

Pamela still feels the need to binge very occasionally, but she usually manages to avoid vomiting afterwards. She says that she is now prepared to take responsibility for what she has eaten, think positively about the food, and accept the consequences of eating it.

Although there is of course a strong psychological element in eating disorders, many experts assume that it is a purely psychological problem, and leave out the possibility of any physical reasons. This diet will not solve your psychological problems for you, but it has a remarkable way of putting them in perspective. If you are a compulsive eater, you will find it a useful and practical way of ending binges and rebuilding your health.

Renee: A reluctant addict

Renee has eczema on her face and in her hair, suffers from palpitations and insomnia, and is ten pounds overweight. Despite all these problems she considers herself to be in good health. She loves 'unhealthy' food, such as cream and white bread, and is generally fond of food, finding it comforting when she is tired or stressed. She tends to change her mood frequently and is quick to take offence. Outwardly she is generous, intelligent and full of life and humour, but inwardly she is agitated and often angry and puzzled by her own unpredictable behaviour.

Most importantly, Renee can't stand health freaks! She finds them annoying because they preach 'healthy eating' at her from some imagined position of superiority. All the foods Renee really loves to eat are supposed to be 'bad for her' and naturally enough she doesn't want to know about 'healthy eating'. Of course she does not yet realise that the Food Addict's Diet is a painless, satisfying and delicious diet change that does not look or feel like a health freak's diet.

If she would only try it, her friends would never guess,

from seeing her eat three good meals a day and snacks whenever she wanted them, that she was on a diet at all!

There is a strong link between food intolerance and mental state, and if Renee were to try it, the Food Addict's Diet could help her by simply calming her enough to see life more clearly and deal with people more patiently. Unfortunately, she is still sceptical. She says that she would rather live with all her problems than face life without her favourite foods. She is an addict, but will not admit it.

I hope, as more and more people try this diet and discover the rewards it can bring, that Renee and all her fellow reluctant food addicts may be encouraged at least to try the experiment. Paradoxically, people who are reluctant to try this diet have the most to gain from it, for they are food addicts, and this is what makes them sceptical. It is good for this group to reserve judgement until they have proved for themselves whether the diet really works. Believe me, it does, sometimes in quite unexpected ways. Give the Food Addict's Diet just three weeks and it could change your whole attitude to yourself and your food!

HOW TO USE THIS BOOK

This book is divided into four parts.

Part One is an introduction to food addiction, and how it has moulded your diet. There is also a great deal to learn about yourself: you will find some charts and quizzes to help you see the present situation with regard to your eating habits and your health.

Part Two gives detailed instructions about the three-week experiment, with menus, tips and advice to help you every step of the way. There is more to learn about yourself, with a second quiz to highlight the many changes that will have taken place in those three short weeks. Here you will find the 'rest test': this will show you the strength of your addiction.

In Part Two, you will find six ways to choose from to accelerate weight loss, if this is what you require.

Part Three gives more detail on the other ways the diet can help you and your family. Here you will find advice for parents and compulsive eaters, and further details for people anxious to discover the cause of their food intolerance symptoms. There is also a section for women, and finally some further information on other addictions, and how they can be brought under control with the help of the Food Addict's Diet.

Finally, there is a recipe section to help you get the most from this diet change, plus some further information for anyone who wants to take things further.

A DIET CHANGE FOR LIFE!

Once you have overcome the effects of food addiction on your diet, you will find you have automatically and easily changed to a healthier way of eating, largely as a result of the foods you have learned to bring in as substitutes for the zero foods. At first they will seem unfamiliar, but soon they will be old friends.

Once you have tried and learned from the Food Addict's Diet, you will find yourself eating more fruit and vegetables, seeds, nuts and breads made from different grains – instead of getting most of your fibre from brown bread and bran. You will obtain protein not only from meat and fish, but nuts, seeds, beans, pulses and whole grains as well. You will be aware of the many sources of calcium: fish, seeds, nuts and green leafy vegetables. All this will have the effect of widening your diet and introducing you to all kinds of food you never thought of using before.

This new way of eating, based on almost 200 natural, whole ingredients eaten at a rate of more than twenty a day, and sometimes as many as fifty in a week, will be the healthiest and most interesting dietary change you ever made in your life.

Part One
You and Your Food

CHAPTER 1
Four Zero Foods

This book is about four particular foods, and their role in our daily diet. They are milk, wheat, potatoes and sugar, and they are about to become our four 'zero' foods.

OVERCOMING OUR ADDICTION TO OUR STAPLE FOODS

The Food Addict's Diet works on a simple principle: that there is a way to overcome any addiction. First, you discover what the culprit is, and then you give it up. In time, the craving for it diminishes and, as long as your intake of it remains carefully controlled, the addiction can be said to have been overcome – though there may be a tendency to lapse from time to time.

It is not difficult to guess the culprits: they are our four favourites, our four staples, and they turn up at almost every meal.

FOUR STAPLE FOODS

In Britain we have a gentle climate that supports a wide range of plant and animal life and, in addition, our trading links around the world guarantee a varied supply of foods all the year round. We have available to us at some stage in the year over 200 basic foods, all reasonably priced and delicious, which you can see listed on pages 95–107.

Despite this, there is a sameness to our daily diet in Britain: every day we eat much the same food, and our shopping baskets tend to contain the same favourites each week. If you glance at any recipe book, you will notice how many dishes are designed to contain some form of milk, wheat, potatoes or sugar. We have become so dependent upon these ingredients that we can hardly imagine a meal without them.

HOW WERE THE FOUR ZEROS CHOSEN?

The magic of the Food Addict's Diet comes from a very simple decision: to remove for three weeks four of our staple foods, and see what happens when we try to live without them. Although when I tried the diet on myself I initially chose the four zeros by guesswork, the success of the diet trials proved that I had guessed correctly.

During the diet trials I questioned all my guinea pigs about their eating habits. All of them said that they consumed wheat and cows' milk in some form every day, and even though many of them did not add sugar to drinks, they still ate it daily – often hidden in processed food. Most of them ate potatoes – or their close relative, the tomato – as a snack, or with their main meal, almost every day.

This result was hardly a surprise: wheat, milk, sugar and potatoes are our staple foods. They are cheap, tasty, versatile and pure, and most people love them. This would not be a problem if we had not based our entire diet upon them to the exclusion of dozens of other foods. Our dependence upon our staples lies at the root of the problem of food addiction: we eat just a few basic food ingredients every day, and even if some of us are not addicted to them, we certainly behave as if we were!

18

CAN I STAY HEALTHY WITHOUT THE FOUR ZEROS?

It would seem from what we hear from the media that milk is our only source of calcium, brown bread our only source of fibre, sugar our only source of energy, and potatoes our only source of complex carbohydrates. This is not so.

In many other countries of the world entire populations live out healthy lives without a single taste of wheat, sugar, potatoes or cow's milk. We are reluctant, almost afraid, to change the way we eat, even though clearly there are many different foods that can be combined to build a perfectly healthy diet. The British diet based on our four staples is not the only healthy diet in the world: in fact, there is increasing evidence that it ranks as one of the unhealthiest.

In 1983 the NACNE (National Advisory Committee on Nutrition Education) report[1] was published after many years of consideration and debate about how to improve our unhealthy British diet. Here are some of the recommendations it contained.

WE MUST EAT THE RIGHT NUMBER OF CALORIES

Most of us need only about 2,500 calories to provide all the energy we need, although needs do vary. The foods that are highest in calories are the starchy, sugary, fatty foods. Sugar, wheat flour and dairy fat are used in most of our most fattening dishes, so giving them up will be a useful way to cut calories, provided, of course, that we replace them with a set of lower-calorie foods. You will find yourself doing that on the Food Addict's Diet, once your addictions are under control.

NOT TOO MUCH SATURATED FAT, MORE UNSATURATED FAT

There are some regularly eaten foods that are high in saturated fat, particularly meats and dairy produce. According to the NACNE report, foods high in saturated fat should be reduced by about 30 per cent and foods containing the other fats should be increased. Dairy products supplied about 30 per cent of the saturated fat in the British diet in 1984.[2] As the Food Addict's Diet cuts out all milk products, the fat content of the diet is cut at a stroke by 30 per cent.

In place of milk, milk-free margarine and oils high in unsaturated fats are used, and oily nuts and seeds, rich in natural unsaturated oils, are highly recommended as a substitute protein, fat and energy source.

LOW IN REFINED CARBOHYDRATES, HIGH IN COMPLEX CARBOHYDRATES

'Refined' carbohydrates mean flours and starches *extracted* from various cereals and starchy root vegetables, and also pure sugar extracted from sugar beet and sugar cane. 'Complex' carbohydrates are starches and sugars that have not been refined – in other words, they remain 'whole'.

Neither wheat nor sugar are allowed on the diet, so at once refined carbohydrates are cut to a minimum. Although no potatoes are allowed, complex carbohydrates are available from other root vegetables and other wholegrain flours, fruits, nuts, beans and seeds. All these are used freely in the Food Addict's Diet as substitutes for the four zero foods.

LESS PROCESSED FOOD GENERALLY

Processed food is limited on this diet for the simple reason that so much of it contains at least one of the zero foods. Also, released from your addictions by the diet, you will rediscover real food, and probably begin to take more interest in cooking using fresh, natural ingredients.

ARE THE ZERO FOODS BAD FOR ME?

No! All four of the zero foods (with the possible exception of sugar) are nutritious and healthy, and eaten in moderation they can contribute a great deal to your diet.

However, cows' milk and wheat have already been found by several allergy experts to be the most likely causes of food intolerance symptoms, and a diet eliminating them completely has already been recommended as a treatment for a wide range of symptoms.[3] If you have a persistent weight or health problem, it is highly likely that you are intolerant to one of the zero foods. If you have eaten it every day of your life you will have spent many years living in a perpetual state of reaction. In that way, one of the four zeros may be 'bad' for you at the moment, but if you take the advice in this book, you may be able to eat it again in the future with no problems.

The four zeros are high in calories, are often taken in a highly refined form, and are so tasty that they are often eaten to excess. Thus they are a problem, but the greatest danger to your health comes from the simple fact that we have based our entire national diet upon them.

Now let's look at each of them in turn, and see how easy it will be to live without them for a while.

GOING AGAINST THE GRAIN (giving up wheat)

WHY GIVE UP WHEAT?

Wheat and excess weight
Addiction to wheat seems to be very common among the overweight. All the foods we make from wheat flour are

high in calories and they are usually restricted in low-calorie diets. Slimmers often break their slimming diet with a wheat-based food. Wheat flour and the foods we make from it seem to be almost irresistible to a hungry slimmer, and they are often used as 'binge' food by compulsive eaters.

Wheat and food intolerance

Wheat is among the top six foods generally considered most likely to cause food intolerance, and I found that several of my candidates on the diet trials reacted to wheat by abdominal bloating and fluid retention.

Wheat flour *seems* to be a pure product. However, traces of chemical residues remain in the flour from insecticides used on the growing plants and fungicides used during storage. As these residues tend to cling to the outer surface of the wheat, they are found in their largest concentrations in the bran, and of course in wholewheat flour.

Some experts suggest that food intolerance is more likely to be the result of these chemical residues than a reaction to the food itself (see pages 180–1). In fact, if you are intolerant of wheat, you may find you are able to tolerate organic wheat flour made from wheat grown without the use of chemicals (but do try the experiment first).

Wheat in disguise

Several people on the trials never realised that they ate wheat many times a day. Read the labels on your packaged food, and discover for yourself the many ways we use wheat. To help you here is a list of disguises.

Flours (self-raising & plain)

White flour, wheatmeal, wholewheat 100% wholemeal (wheat flour is found in most 'Lean Cuisine' dishes); semolina; cracked wheat; bulgar wheat; couscous.

Wheatgerm

As powder (Bemax); in breakfast cereals; wheatgerm oil.

Wheat bran
Raw; included in bran cereal (e.g. All Bran, Farmhouse Bran, Sainsbury's Porridge with Added Bran).

All bakery products (except rye, barley or corn bread)
Breads and rolls; croissants; pastry; cakes.

Slimming breads (e.g. Nimble)

Pizza

Crispbreads
(e.g. Grissini, Cracker Bread, Gourmet Thins, Krackawheat, Scooples); wholemeal bran biscuits; sesame crackers; melba toasts; French toast.

All types of cake mix

Wafers and cones for ice cream

Pastry
Vol au vents; sweet pastries; savoury pies.

Biscuits
Sweet; cheese; cocktail biscuits; cream crackers, etc.

Wholewheat breakfast cereals
Shredded Wheat, Force Wheat Flakes, Weetabix, Shreddies, Puffed Wheat, Sultana Bran, Ready Brek, Jordan's Crispy Muesli, Cinnamon Toast Crunch, Start, Cruesli, Grapenuts, Fruit 'n' Fibre, Sugar Puffs. (Wheat is almost always present in mixed-grain breakfast cereals.)

Rolled whole wheat flakes
In muesli, Jordan's Crunchy Bars.

Rusk
In sausages.

Pasta
Lasagne, cannelloni, spaghetti, macaroni, vermicelli, tagliatelli, etc.

Batter
Around fish, fish fingers and fish cakes; fritters; Yorkshire pudding; pancakes.

Noodles

Stuffing

Taramasalata (in the breadcrumbs)

Fish paste

Croutons

Snacks
Wheat snacks; Twiglets; Mignons Morceaux; various packaged cocktail snacks.

Drinks
Often added to other grains in the manufacture of whisky, whisky liqueurs, gin, vodka, beer, lager.

THE GOODNESS OF WHEAT

Wheat *can* be good for you, if you know how to control it! Wheat flour is ground from the seeds of the wheat plant, which contain all the nutrients the new plant needs to grow. When you eat freshly ground wholewheat, you eat them too; however, if the flour is sifted to remove the bran and the germ to make white flour, much of the goodness disappears.

Untouched wholewheat grains contain Vitamins B1, B2, B5, B6, B3 and D, as well as folic acid, iron, calcium, potassium, magnesium, zinc, copper, chromium, Vitamin E and biotin; and as wheat is a seed, the germ contains several important fatty acids. Wholewheat grains are very hard, and do not soften much even after several hours of boiling, so we make raw wholewheat edible by grinding it into wholewheat flour, puffing it into breakfast cereal, or rolling it into flat flakes.

If wheat is made into 100 per cent wholewheat products, most of the goodness is retained, so when you do try wheat-based foods again once the experiment is over, remember always to use 100 per cent wholemeal flour and avoid products using white flour wherever possible.

CAN WE REMAIN HEALTHY WITHOUT WHEAT?

Wholewheat flour can be an important source of B vitamins, carbohydrate and fibre, but if you do not like wholewheat flour, and always eat your wheat as white flour, then you are not missing much by not eating wheat.

If you have been used to taking all your wheat flour wholemeal and stoneground, or using bran or wheatgerm as a supplement, then when you give up wheat you must find another source of those nutrients from the foods you are allowed to eat (see page 95).

Replacing the B vitamins
The best sources of B vitamins apart from wheat are the other cereals: corn, rice, rye, barley and oats, so the simplest way to replace wheat is to use foods using these cereals – such as porridge oats for breakfast, rye crispbread or rice cakes for lunch, and cornflour to thicken the gravy for dinner.

Even so, these other cereals are not essential, as small amounts of the various B vitamins can be found in almost all foods.

Here are some of the best sources from those other foods:

B1 (thiamine): nuts and seeds (especially sunflower seeds), seaweed, most vegetables and pork.

B2 (riboflavin): liver, heart and kidney, yeast, pulses, leafy green vegetables, fish, eggs.

B5 (pantothenic acid): offal, peanuts, meat, green vegetables.

B6 (pyridoxine): seeds, yeast, offal, cabbage, eggs and beef.

B3 (niacin): meat, nuts.

(*Source*: Earl Mindell, *The Vitamin Bible* (Arlington Books, 1987).

Replacing the fibre

A high-fibre diet is healthy, for fibre helps to reduce cholesterol levels and prevent bowel disorders and constipation. Many people think that wheatbran is the only source of fibre, with oatbran a close second: it isn't. The outer skins of all the various wholegrains are high in fibre, and if you eat any other wholegrain cereal or wholegrain flour you will be eating fibre. A packet of oatbran costs twice as much as a packet of porridge oats, but the whole oats still have their bran wrapped around them, and taste much better!

All plant food contains fibre: you don't need bran. To guarantee a good fibre intake make sure that you eat plenty of foods that comes from plants: beans, seeds, roots, stems, leaves or even flowers! (See the 200 allowed foods on page 101.)

LIVING WITHOUT WHEAT

The last slice of cake does not tempt you, and biscuits go soggy in the tin for want of someone to eat them. You nibble daintily on a rye crispbread, keeping your dieting intentions intact.

Your 'bread and spread' habit has ended and other exciting grain-based dishes have entered your daily fare (see recipe section on pages 245–85 for details). All grains are eaten whole or as a wholegrain flour, and the amount of fibre and B vitamins in your diet has increased, bringing an end to constipation.

All this can be possible when you give up wheat on the Food Addict's Diet.

LOSING YOUR BOTTLE (giving up milk)

IMPORTANT NOTE:

If you believe you may suffer from food intolerance of any kind, or have allergies, then take care! The zero foods experiment could be the first time in your whole life that you have lived longer than two or three days without milk. In the first few weeks before overcoming your addiction, you may be extremely sensitive to the smallest amount, so be careful while you are on the plan that you do not take any milk or milk products by mistake, or you may be in for a very bad attack of your usual symptoms.

WHY GIVE IT UP?

Milk and excess weight
On any slimming diet we are warned against full-cream milk, and told that we must take our milk skimmed, our yoghurt low-fat, and avoid completely cream and condensed milk. The zero plan cuts out *all* the fat and calories in milk, by simply cutting out milk itself.

Milk and food intolerance
The human is the only animal on earth to drink milk as an adult as part of its regular diet. Some people cannot take milk because they lack the necessary enzyme to digest it (this enzyme is called lactase). If you are a member of an African, Oriental or Asian race, there is a good chance that you are lactase deficient. According to Leon Chaitow in his book *Stone Age Diet* (Optima, 1987), 90 per cent of the world's population could be lactase deficient, and that probably includes you! Lactase deficiency usually manifests itself as persistent diarrhoea, flatulence, stomach pain or other digestive disturbances, and these clear up

27

very quickly once all milk products are removed from the diet.

Milk is capable of carrying residues of chemicals on the grass or fodder that makes up the cow's diet, as well as hormones given to increase milk yield. If you decide to return to using milk products again after trying the experiment, I recommend that you start using organically produced milk.

Milk in disguise

Notice in your recipe books how many recipes require some kind of milk product. Even if you never drink liquid milk, you are probably eating it in several other forms:

Liquid milk
Whole milk; homogenised milk; semi-skimmed milk; skimmed milk; sterilised milk ('Long Life'); condensed milk; evaporated milk.

High-fat milk products:
Cream; soured cream; butter.

Milk solids
Junket (milk set with rennet); yoghurt.

Cheeses
Hard cheese; curd cheese; cottage cheese; Quark; Fromage Frais; processed cheese; cheese spreads.

Added to processed foods
Soft cheese (in fish pâtés); hard cheese (in cheese biscuits and cocktail snacks); yoghurt (in tzatziki); milk solids (in milk chocolate and other confectionery); whey powder (in margarine); dried milk powder (in biscuits, cakes, cake mixes, dessert mixes, etc.); lactic acid (in coleslaw and prepared salads); casein (in soups, stews and savoury ready-prepared foods).

THE GOODNESS OF MILK

Milk is an important source of protein, calories, saturated fat, Vitamin D, calcium and riboflavin (Vitamin B2).

At one time the protein and energy in milk kept our city populations from starvation, but milk is not now of such importance as a source of protein, except possibly among people on very low incomes. Today, cows' milk is considered primarily as an important source of calcium in our diet, essential for healthy bones and teeth.

CAN WE REMAIN HEALTHY WITHOUT MILK?

Millions of people living healthily in Japan and parts of China do not keep cows (or any other animals) for their milk, and in fact do not use milk at all.

Replacing the saturated fat
Whole milk is high in saturated fat, which we should avoid to maintain good health. A statistical link has been found between death from coronary heart disease and the consumption of cows' milk, particularly among men aged 55–64. This link was also clear when the consumption of milk protein was considered even without the fat.[4]

Replacing the Vitamin D in milk
Without sufficient Vitamin D in your diet, you cannot properly absorb calcium from your food. However, most Vitamin D is made in the skin in the presence of sunlight, so it is important to go out in daylight every day. A lack of Vitamin D can cause rickets, especially among dark-skinned people in this country.

Vitamin D is found in small quantities in deep-sea fish-liver oils, sardines, herring, salmon and tuna, and tiny amounts are even available from wheatgerm and bacon and eggs.[5] Do be careful of Vitamin D supplements, though, because an excess of this vitamin can be harmful.

Replacing the calcium in milk

Milk provides most of the calcium in the normal British diet, and many people are worried when they decide to avoid milk because of allergy or intolerance that they may become deficient in calcium.

The British Recommended Daily Allowances (RDA) for calcium are 600–700 mg per day for children and teen-agers, and 500 mg per day for adults (1,200 mg per day for women during pregnancy or lactation). However, RDAs vary around the world, so that, for instance, a twenty-five-year-old man apparently only needs 450 mg if he lives in Venezuela, but if he moves to Bulgaria, he will be told he needs almost three times as much – 1,100 mg.[6] There is obviously much confusion about how much calcium we need!

In 1984 dairy products supplied about 500 mg of calcium to the average British diet, and this is what you must replace when you give up milk. Cows' milk is such a rich source of calcium that a pint a day will provide an entire day's supply, so ordinarily it is unnecessary to look for a good calcium supply from other foods. Consequently, few people know where else calcium is to be found.

Generally speaking, the richest sources of calcium are, in order of importance, seeds, fish, nuts, milks (including goats' and sheep's), dark-green leafy vegetables such as watercress or broccoli, dried fruit, wholegrains, beans and pulses – so there are plenty of alternative sources of calcium. If you are particularly concerned about calcium intake, turn to page 286 where I have drawn up a 'Calci-Counter' of our favourite foods; this will help you when you go shopping.

In the early days of the diet I would suggest taking a calcium tablet of about 500 mg every day until you have adjusted your diet to include plenty of calcium-rich, non-milk products. Some high-quality mineral waters contain high levels of calcium, and people who live in hard-water areas can obtain calcium from their cooking and drinking water;[7] softening or filtering water removes much of its calcium.

Replacing the protein in milk

Low-fat cheese, low-fat yoghurt and skimmed milk have become popular protein foods. When you replace them in your new diet you will have to think of other protein foods that can be used in a similar way: replace cheese with pâté or hummus (for ideas, see recipes, page 249), replace yoghurt with a soya dessert, and instead of skimmed milk use a nut milk (see recipes, page 245).

Milk is a cheap source of protein, and you may think that alternatives will be expensive. If you are on a tight budget, use beans and seeds as an alternative source of cheap protein. In the recipe section you will find ideas for soups, main meals and dips using beans and seeds.

LIVING WITHOUT MILK

Some of us have strong emotions about milk: we think of it as a 'complete' food that contains all that is needed for life, no doubt thinking of the days when our mother's milk was our only food. We associate it with contented cows grazing in country meadows in summertime.

Tea or coffee can taste good without milk. Try herb teas or China tea if you find ordinary tea too bitter without it. For some people, black coffee is an acquired taste, but it is very refreshing. Remember that if you take drinks such as tea or coffee without milk they contain no calories at all!

If you spread butter and cheese on bread every day and call it 'lunch', you are in for a few surprises when you try the Food Addict's Diet. When you take away that 'prop' of bread and cheese you will discover all kinds of new ideas for quick lunches: more varied, less boring, and much healthier too!

A LUMP IN THE THROAT (giving up sugar)

NOTE: While you are on the Food Addict's Diet you are only going to avoid sugar that comes directly from sugar cane or sugar beet.

WHY GIVE UP SUGAR?

Sugar and excess weight

Sugar is the most addictive of the zero foods. Sugar addicts eat too many sweet foods, gain weight, rot their teeth, spend a great deal of money on confectionery, and in extreme cases may even develop diabetes. Even the mildest sugar addict is likely to break the rules of his slimming diet when confronted by his favourite sweet food.

Most of us can easily maintain our slimming intentions during our main course, but we tend to yield to temptation when it comes to dessert. Sugar itself may not directly affect your weight, but your sugar addiction certainly will!

Sugar and food intolerance

Sugar is not usually named as a major culprit in food intolerance, but high intakes do require massive hormone adjustments, and put a strain on your body's coping system.

Food intolerance arises as a physical reaction to overdose. Sugar is so pure and concentrated that it is very easy to overdose, and it tastes so good that we often do! Each time you overdose on sugar your pancreas has to produce massive doses of insulin to prevent your blood sugar from becoming too high. So if you ever find yourself eating a whole packet of sweets at one go, think of the work you are giving your pancreas!

Sugar in disguise

Beet and cane sugar have many different names. Here is a list of the sugars that are not allowed on the Food Addict's Diet:

Granulated sugar; icing sugar; brown sugar (demerara, muscovado); molasses; raw cane sugar; beet sugar; cane sugar; block sugar; preserving sugar; caster sugar; golden syrup; black treacle.

Sugar can come in various disguises, and have many

other names. You may see some of them on the labels of packeted foods, but not realise that they are sugars. Those to avoid are:

Sucrose
Just another name for sugar.

Glucose
You can buy this as a powder or as sweets for extra energy.

Glucose syrup
Usually found in sweets and confectionery.

Dextrose
Sugar used as a preservative in preserved meats such as ham.

You may occasionally see *lactose* (milk sugar) or *high fructose syrup* as an ingredient in your food: these are to be avoided too.

THE GOODNESS OF SUGAR

Sugar has no food value at all, although brown sugar, molasses and black treacle do contain small amounts of the B vitamins. Sugar gives energy, and most of the advertising claims about sugar mention its taste or the energy it gives. In fact, sugar gives you no more energy than the other carbohydrate foods.

Sugar gives you calories and nothing else. Sweet food is tempting and easy to overeat, and acts against a healthy diet by pushing other more nutritious food aside – unless you have an appetite big enough to take sugary snacks and still manage a balanced diet besides!

CAN WE REMAIN HEALTHY WITHOUT SUGAR?

Your body simply does not need sugar and you could live the rest of your life without it and come to no harm at all.

Replacing the energy

At first, food addicts who have made sugar a major part of their diet will miss those calories! If you are fat this is good news, but if you are thin, this may make you thinner, so eat plenty of other energy-giving foods, such as dates, figs and other dried fruits, and starchy foods made from grains, beans and root vegetables. You will soon gain weight again.

Replacing the taste

There are a variety of substitutes for sugar, including honey and maple syrup. While on the diet you can enjoy corn sugar (sorbitol) in 'sugar-free' sweets, or use fructose crystals in just the same way that you would use granulated sugar.

Could you live without sugar?

The results of the 1988 diet trials were interesting: although sugar addiction is the most widely recognised form of food addiction, only 22 per cent found sugar 'very difficult' to give up, but 54 per cent had problems giving up milk. The majority of those who claimed, before starting the diet, that sugar was their 'real problem', were surprised at how quickly their sugar cravings died during the experiment.

In the first few days of the experiment you may feel a need for sweetness: make sure you have bought enough dried fruits (dates and figs are good) and other sweeteners that will satisfy your cravings (see pages 282–4 for other ideas).

Once you are free of your craving for sugar you can look forward to discovering the real taste of some of your foods and drinks, without the mask of added sugar. You will find new sweeteners and enjoy new kinds of high-energy snacks. Also, you will soon experience that wonderful feeling of virtue when, without any effort of will, you refuse that tempting piece of chocolate and keep your slimming diet intact!

WHEN YOU HAVE HAD YOUR CHIPS (giving up potatoes)

WHY GIVE UP POTATOES?

Potatoes and excess weight

Potatoes are not very high in calories (a boiled potato contains 22 calories per ounce), but we love to eat fat with them. We put butter and cheese on our jacket potatoes, add butter and milk to our mashed potato, and add fat from the joint to roast potatoes. Our favourite way to eat potatoes is as chips and crisps, which are cooked in oil. When potatoes cooked in this way are excluded from your diet, a great many calories and fat units will go with them!

Potatoes and food intolerance

Potatoes contain several alkaloids, drug-like chemicals found in various plants that have a noticeable effect on the nervous system. Among the alkaloids found in potatoes is solanine, found mostly just under the skin. The flesh of a normal healthy potato contains only between 1 and 5 mg of solanine per 100 g, but there is rather more in the skin and the eye (30–50 mg per 100 g).[8] This means that those who seek extra vitamins and fibre by eating the skin will eat more solanine.

Solanine is poisonous in large amounts. Levels of more than 30 mg of solanine per 100 mg can cause digestive disorders and even hallucinations.[9] Potatoes develop more solanine in response to damage or sunlight, so never eat damaged or green potatoes.

Intolerance to potatoes is quite common, and worth considering if you have a weight or health problem. As children eat so many potatoes in the form of crisps and chips, it is worth considering whether your child is intolerant to them. (Special advice for parents can be found in Chapter 14.)

Potatoes in disguise

Potatoes appear in our lives in many forms, such as: crisps; potato snacks (Hula Hoops, Wotsits, Monster

Munchs, etc.); potato chips; jacket potatoes; potato starch/flour (can be bought in health-food shops); as an ingredient of prepared frozen meals.

They also come hidden in other foods. Read the labels on your food and you will soon see how often potatoes are used in processed foods, such as: fish cakes; canned foods (e.g. soups, salads, mixed vegetables, stews); Cornish pasties; meat and vegetable pies.

THE GOODNESS OF POTATOES

Like all other root vegetables, potatoes are a storehouse of energy, vitamins and minerals. They provide starch and vegetable protein, Vitamins B1, B2, B3 and C, and iron, phosphorus, calcium and potassium.

Most of the nutrients are found just under the skin, which itself contains most of the potassium, so potato flour or snacks made only from the flesh do not contain these nutrients. Potatoes must be cooked whole to obtain all this goodness, but do remember that most of the solanine in potatoes is also found in the skin or just under it.

CAN WE REMAIN HEALTHY WITHOUT POTATOES?

Potatoes are only one kind of starchy root vegetable, and there are plenty of alternatives – such as swedes, turnips, carrots, parsnips, sweet potatoes, or even yams! (see recipes on pages 248–9 for more detail.)

Replacing the starch
On the Food Addict's Diet you can obtain your starches from breads and crispbreads made with non-wheat flour, and other starchy foods, such as millet and rice, can be a tasty alternative with a main meal.

Replacing the fibre

The Food Addict's Diet is a high-fibre diet, so you have no need to worry about being short of fibre as long as you keep up your consumption of fruits and vegetables.

Could you live without potatoes?

In your search for potato alternatives you will have to start using other root vegetables, and you will find yourself cooking three or four different vegetables with a main meal instead of just 'spuds and one other'. Look out for old English traditional recipes using other starch foods: dishes invented long before the days when no meal was considered complete without potatoes.

When you are looking for a snack in the pub, ask the barman for raw peanuts with raisins instead of crisps, and take a little more time preparing packed lunches, finding other foods to replace the old standbys like crisps.

THREE EXTRA ZEROS

WHAT ARE THEY?

The three extra zeros are:

1. Tomatoes (raw, cooked and processed into sauces, flavourings, etc.).
2. Aubergines.
3. All kinds of peppers: green, red, chilli, paprika, hot, sweet and so on, except for black and white pepper.

The nightshade family

Potatoes, tomatoes, aubergines and all kinds of peppers are members of the same family: the *solanacae* or nightshade-plant family. They all contain alkaloids, which are poisonous in large amounts. The most poisonous member of this family is belladonna, or deadly nightshade.

When I started to research the effects of potatoes, it became clear that each one of the nightshade family contains an alkaloid of some kind.

37

WHY GIVE UP THESE THREE EXTRA ZEROS?

Alkaloids and addictions

We saw on page 35 how the presence of solanine in potatoes is probably the reason why people become addicted to them and develop symptoms of food intolerance as a result: the alkaloids in any of the other nightshades can have a similar effect.

Most highly addictive drugs, such as morphine and its derivatives, caffeine (in coffee and tea) and theobromine (in cocoa), are alkaloids. They have quite pronounced physical and mental effects, and are highly addictive. In Chapter 10 we will look at how you can extend the Food Addict's Diet to include three extra zeros (tomatoes, peppers and aubergines) in order to reduce your dependence on tea, coffee, chocolate or cigarettes.

Exactly when you take this step is up to you: I would suggest that if you think just four zero foods is enough to start with, then leave the three extra zeros until later, after the three-week experiment. However, if you want to achieve maximum results in the minimum time, avoid all seven zero foods right from the start. You will notice when you come to the list of 200 allowed foods on page 98 that all seven zero foods are missing.

Nightshades: the world's most popular food

It seems that the slightly addictive quality of the nightshade family of vegetables has guaranteed their success worldwide. The taste of tomato with peppers has become the hallmark of Italian food, and of all the European traditional diets that have been exported along with the pioneers, Italian recipes based on tomatoes and peppers have become most in demand.

The pizza is now more popular than the hamburger as the worldwide fast-food favourite, and it is easy to see why. On each pizza there is an irresistible combination of our most addictive favourite foods: grilled cheese, tomato and peppers, resting on a circle of crisp freshly baked bread made from wheat flour.

FOUR ZERO FOODS

So now you know a little more about the four foods that underpin the diet of every Western country of the world. Once these four foods were only minor additions to the diet, but today they penetrate into every meal and snack we eat. Later on we will see how our love for them has produced our narrow and repetitive diet, and underlies a great many of our problems with food.

The four zeros are all natural and nutritious foods, and are not harmful or unhealthy. The problem is simply that we eat too much of them. This is not just because they are cheap and easy to obtain: eating them gives us pleasure, no meal feels complete without them, and some of us cannot live without just a little of each of them every day. In short, we are addicted to them.

In the next few chapters I hope to break down a few more myths about you and your food. I will show you how our so-called 'healthy and varied' diet is a myth, that you are not always as healthy as you make out, and that your personal diet is rather repetitive. Running as a thread through these three chapters will be the idea of food addiction.

Are you a food addict? To follow the Food Addict's Diet you will have to live without the four zero foods completely, and if the mere thought of doing this fills you with horror, you need look no further for proof: you are a food addict! Later in Part Two I will not only reveal your addiction to you, but also provide a simple, cheap and natural way to overcome it. Once this has happened you will find a wonderful new range of foods opening up before you to use in building yourself a totally new kind of diet.

CHAPTER 2
You and Your Health

You are about to try the zero foods experiment, which I hope will bring about several important changes in your health and diet. In order to see these changes clearly, though, we must first assess the present situation. You then try the experiment, and after that take another look at how things stand.

This chapter looks first at you, and how you feel both physically and mentally. Chapter 3 will look at the place of food and drink in your life, and Chapter 4 will show you how to make a food diary, to find out exactly what food ingredients you are using. In this way the three chapters will help you to obtain a complete picture of where you are today in relation to your food.

HOW ARE YOU?

If you have only a few minor symptoms, then probably when people ask you how you are, you say, 'I'm fine!' But are you really?

Are you healthy?
Underline the statement that applies to you: I am very healthy/I am in reasonable health/I have some health

problems/I have some major health problems/I feel ill most of the time.*

(*If you underlined this response, make sure that your doctor knows that you intend to try a change of diet so that he can monitor your progress.)

Do you ever have attacks of any of these symptoms?
(Circle 'yes' if you do, and 'no' if you don't.)

Nose and chest
(other than when you have a cold or infection)

persistent runny nose	yes/no
persistent catarrh	yes/no
persistent dry cough	yes/no
sneezing	yes/no
sore throat	yes/no
wheezing	yes/no
hay fever	yes/no
mouth ulcers	yes/no
sinusitis	yes/no

Eyes

dark rings around eyes	yes/no
'bags' under eyes	yes/no
red itchy eyes	yes/no

Ears

red ear	yes/no
itching in the ear	yes/no
noises in the ear	yes/no
dizziness	yes/no

Hair

dry scaly scalp	yes/no
dandruff	yes/no
itchy scalp	yes/no

Pulse
rapid heartbeat   yes/no
irregular heartbeat   yes/no

Circulation
faintness   yes/no
unreasonable feeling of cold   yes/no
unreasonable feeling of heat   yes/no

Lungs
asthma   yes/no
hyperventilation (overbreathing)   yes/no

Digestion
nausea or vomiting   yes/no
frequent belching   yes/no
indigestion   yes/no
abdominal bloating   yes/no
alternating constipation and very
  loose motions   yes/no
excessive flatulence   yes/no
acid stomach   yes/no
constipation   yes/no
frequent episodes of diarrhoea   yes/no
bad breath (halitosis)   yes/no
irritable bowel syndrome   yes/no
haemorrhoids   yes/no

Skin
redness   yes/no
acne   yes/no
dry scaly skin   yes/no
rashes   yes/no
eczema   yes/no
hives   yes/no
psoriasis   yes/no
itching without rash   yes/no
blotches   yes/no
excessive sweating   yes/no

Muscles and bones

aching joints	yes/no
aching muscles	yes/no
swollen joints	yes/no
stiffness	yes/no
backache	yes/no
tremor of the hands, head, etc.	yes/no
stiff neck	yes/no

Urinary

fluid retention (puffy ankles and face)	yes/no
excessive urine production	yes/no
scanty urine production	yes/no

Head

migraine	yes/no
throbbing	yes/no
headaches	yes/no

Women's problems

menstrual difficulties	yes/no
thrush	yes/no

Make a list of those symptoms that you experience most often. You will be asked again about your own list of current symptoms in Chapter 7.

My minor symptoms at present are:

....
....
....
....

Learning to live with it

If you have ringed 'yes' for any of these symptoms, you probably suffer from occasional attacks that fade away, only to come back when you least expect it. Alternatively, you may suffer all day every day, but you are never *really* ill because of it. People are reluctant to go to

43

the doctor with minor symptoms, because they are not ill and would feel like a malingerer if they went to the surgery. They are most likely to mention symptoms 'by the way' when attending the surgery for a more pressing problem.

Some of these problems are persistent, defying all attempts at treatment for many years. Some treatments may work for a time, but often they cease to be effective. Sometimes treatment does not help at all; and as there is nothing that can be done, you are told that you must 'learn to live with it'.

That is easy to say. These symptoms can become a terrible drain on your energy, and even be quite disabling. A bad rash on your face, for example, can make you feel disfigured, and aching joints can make you disinclined to walk in the fresh air, simply because it hurts to do so.

'Learning to live with it' usually means keeping quiet about it. If you do have occasional strange attacks of something like faintness or rapid heartbeat, you are unlikely to mention it, as the feeling quickly passes and it may never happen again. If you do tell your doctor, and he finds nothing physically wrong, he may suggest that it was 'nerves' or 'stress'. So you keep quiet, and do not tell anyone that you perhaps burst into tears when alone at home, or wake in the night convinced that you are about to die, or that you feel sleepy all day and some days your brain feels as if it is disconnected from your body.

A way out
As people on my trials have discovered, food intolerance may be the cause of many of these minor ailments, and the zero foods experiment will help you to discover if you too can gain relief. Several people on the trials were surprised to find that their need for pain killers for headache, arthritis and muscular aches and pains was greatly reduced once they were on the Food Addict's Diet.

Doreen, one of my first candidates, discovered a very strong relationship between wheat and her arthritis pain.

44

She was addicted to bread, and so in the early months of trying to give up wheat she lapsed several times. Every time she managed to give up wheat for a while, her pain eased and her consumption of pain killers fell, but as soon as she lapsed and ate bread on a regular basis again, the pain returned with a vengeance. She has now managed to break her addiction entirely, and her requirement for pain killers is now about one-third of what it was before she began the diet.

Clearly, all illness cannot be put down to food intolerance: there are many other possible causes for your symptoms. You may in fact not be intolerant to your food at all, but just reacting to a bad, repetitive diet. Perhaps your problem is simply due to a nutritional deficiency. The object of this diet change is not only to overcome food addiction, but also to create a varied new diet. This is the only sure way to better health, whatever your problem may be.

Keep your doctor informed

If your doctor cannot find out what is wrong, perhaps another doctor can, so do ask.

Unfortunately, professional advice about the diagnosis and treatment of food intolerance is very limited, except in the field of alternative medicine. Some health professionals believe that experimenting with the diet is dangerous, and that people may imagine that some foods are 'making them ill'.

Consequently, some patients may try self-treatment for illness by altering their diet and avoiding going to their doctor. In some cases, this course of action could mean that a serious illness remains undiagnosed.

This is why I recommend that you take this book to your doctor and tell him that you intend to change your diet to relieve your symptoms. Later on, you could send him a note or tell him about your progress, for if your symptoms do improve he should be told. If more and more patients talked to their doctors in this way about how their health is being affected by their food, the need for properly regulated NHS treatment for food allergy and intolerance could one day be recognised and met.

Trust your own judgement
Although I recommend keeping your doctor informed of your progress, only you, by learning to listen to your body's needs, will be able to tell if this diet change helps you to feel better. Your body has an enormous ability to heal itself, but first you must create the right conditions for healing with a good, varied diet.

MIND AND BODY

The state of your mind and your body are bound together. Your attitude to both yourself and your food problem can be coloured by your mental state, and your mental state may actually be affected by the foods you eat. Various forms of mental illness have been related to food intolerance by several experts, including Dr Richard Mackarness, who rocked the medical and psychiatric world in 1976 with his book *Not All in the Mind*. This book has become a classic text for those seeking alternative cures for mental illness.

So, in the light of this idea, let's take a look at your state of mind at the moment. You may find some changes in your mood after you start the diet, and it will be useful to compare this with your present state. You will be asked to refer to this chart again when we reach Chapter 7.

Assessing your mental state
Do you have occasional attacks of any of the following? If so, circle 'yes'.

feeling stressed	yes/no
lack of confidence	yes/no
episodes of depression	yes/no
mild anxiety state	yes/no

constant nervousness	yes/no
occasional panic attacks	yes/no
insomnia	yes/no
episodes of hyperactivity	yes/no
frequent nervous exhaustion	yes/no
irritability	yes/no
occasional inability to think clearly	yes/no
brain 'fag'	yes/no
trembling	yes/no
lightheadedness	yes/no

If you have circled 'yes' against any of these, it may be that food intolerance is the cause of the problem. Specific foods have been implicated in mental symptoms – particularly milk, wheat, sugar and caffeine drinks.[1]

During the diet trials there was a noticeable change of mood, even among those who were obviously rather highly strung individuals. Many of the candidates said that they were sleeping better and felt more rested, and all of them felt their mood lift as their energy increased.

The real test came when their three-week commitment ended, and most of them returned to eating their favourite foods again. A long-term follow-up showed that both their physical and mental state had reverted to how it was before they began the diet.

Rosemary learns to beat despair

Rosemary applied to join the trials as needing to lose weight, but her greatest problem was a 'workaholic' husband; she felt abandoned by him and left to shoulder the burden of the family. Rosemary was very depressed, and described herself as suicidal. After less than a week on the diet she no longer felt her husband was neglecting her, but instead felt sure that he was building up a business for the benefit of the family as a whole.

The marital tension eased for the next six months as she continued her slimming effort on the diet. Eventually the summer holidays came and, in the manner of all food addicts, Rosemary gave in once more to her addiction for chocolate and pasta. She was plunged into an almost suicidal despair almost immediately.

Eventually I made contact with her and promised her a more positive mood if she would begin the diet again. Within a week she was much happier and busy again, only to be plunged into despair when she lapsed once more. We have repeated this cycle again and again over the last three years. Now she has learned to overcome her addiction, and has discovered through her many failures the link between particular foods, her attitude, and her state of mind.

She now knows that certain foods (chocolate and wheat) are better avoided altogether. She is now so busy dashing about involved in school activities with the children that she seems to have forgotten that her husband was ever a problem. He is still a workaholic, but Rosemary now has the confidence and energy to build a good life for herself at home. Recently she joined a slimming club, determined that she would stick with a diet through thick and thin and win her husband back to her side with a new trim figure. She has lost two stones already, but she does not seem to have noticed that her happier mood has done more for the marriage than a new figure could ever do!

Stress

Stress is such a prevalent problem today that we are often unaware of the stresses we undergo. Almost everyone in modern life is under stress of some sort but, regardless of how much stress there is on you, you should be able to find a way of coping with it. Coping with stress requires energy and confidence. An extraordinary effect of the Food Addict's Diet is that it increases both.

MORE ENERGY FOR LIFE

This is the greatest reward that this diet change will bring you, and by the end of your first week on the diet you will find yourself feeling more active and alive. So that you will be able to see this change clearly, note below what your present level of energy is (underline the one that applies to you):

Level 1: constantly tired and lacking in energy
Level 2: lack energy most of the time
Level 3: usually have enough energy for my way of life
Level 4: normally quite energetic
Level 5: abounding energy

On page 127 you will be asked the same question again, and you will be able to see then how much your energy level has been raised.

Sandra: Tired of life

Here is an example of someone whose life was completely transformed by the extra energy this diet change has given her; this was my first report on Sandra when she applied to join the trials:

'Sandra is a housewife at home with two small children, both attending nursery school. For most of the day she has to fight a strong desire to fall asleep in order to finish her housework. Sometimes she just sits and stares out of the window with her mind a blank.

'At breakfast time she is never hungry, and the very thought of food makes her feel ill, but by ten o'clock she is ready to eat the contents of the biscuit tin with two cups of hot milky coffee and two sugars. This snack usually acts as a stimulant to help her to begin the housework at last. Lunch for Sandra is another snack plus the children's left-overs. In the afternoon a friend sometimes drops in and out comes another packet of biscuits.

'Teatime means another guilty nibble (left-overs again) and then that endless hungry wait before supper with Jim who usually likes a steak or a grill with chips. Sandra usually finds that she has nibbled enough through the day to keep going without eating a "big meal". In fact, she now finds that if she eats a large supper late at night she feels uncomfortably bloated.

'Since her last pregnancy she has been seven pounds overweight, and has a wardrobe full of lovely clothes that no longer fit.

'Sandra never eats breakfast, rarely eats lunch, and eats fresh vegetables hardly at all. She hates salads, and only likes carrots. She loves chips and toast. She admits that she cannot resist a packet of biscuits once it has been opened, and she sometimes drinks ten cups of coffee in a day. She could not be eating a worse diet if she tried. Not only is she eating all four zeros at virtually every meal, but she is eating hardly anything else.'

Sandra tries the diet:
Starting the diet was a big step for Sandra, but she began to feel its benefits long before she had lost a single pound. Within two weeks her energy began to increase. She found herself cleaning the garage out in the afternoon of the second Tuesday on the diet, and the next Friday she felt alert enough to take the children to the park. That weekend she made her first special effort with the family lunchtime meal: she made a finger salad with dips, which they all enjoyed – even the children.

She has now redecorated the living room on her own, and is redesigning the garden to grow her own vegetables. She is one of my most able evangelists, and she is of course no longer tired.

YOU AND YOUR WEIGHT

How overweight are you?
I think my ideal weight is . . . . . st . . . . . lb (. . . . kg)
I am . . . . in (. . . . . cm) tall.

To give you an idea of how much you should weigh, look up your height on the chart.

Men

Height without shoes

in	cm	Healthy weight range lb	kg
62	158	112–141	51–64
63	160	115–144	52–65
64	163	118–148	54–67
65	165	121–152	55–69
66	168	124–156	56–71
67	170	128–161	58–73
68	173	132–166	60–75
69	175	136–170	62–77
70	178	140–174	64–79
71	180	144–179	65–81
72	183	148–184	67–84
73	185	152–189	69–86
74	188	156–194	71–88
75	191	160–199	73–90
76	193	164–204	74–92

Women

Height without shoes

in	cm	Healthy weight range lb	kg
58	147	92–119	42–54
59	150	94–122	43–55
60	152	96–125	44–57
61	155	99–128	45–58
62	158	102–131	46–59
63	160	105–134	48–61
64	163	108–138	49–63
65	165	111–142	50–64
66	168	114–146	52–66
67	170	118–150	54–68
68	173	122–154	55–70
69	175	126–158	57–72
70	178	130–163	59–74
71	180	134–168	61–76
72	183	138–173	63–78

(Adapted from BUPA leaflet, 'Obesity', BUPA Medical Centre, 1985.)

Being your ideal weight is probably less important than how you look and what clothing size fits you. It has more to do with how you feel than how you look, and of course it has a great deal to do with how you eat. I will ask you again in Chapter 7 if you have lost weight during the experiment, but I hope you are beginning to see that this book is more than a way of changing the number on the scales. We are looking at the very reason why you became overweight in the first place: food addiction.

WHEN DID YOU FIRST GAIN WEIGHT?

There are three kinds of overweight, and the way you see your problem at present will bear some relation to this.

Lifelong overweight
This means that there has never been a time in your life when you have not been fat. If this is so, you probably see being overweight as part of your basic personality, and you simply cannot imagine being any other shape. Dieting for this group means fighting their image of themselves, and every time weight is lost they tend to regain it and return to the same high weight, where they feel normal.

I believe that people in this group are intolerant to foods they were fed in the first days of their life: sugar, cows' milk, wheat and sugar in particular. Until they realise and come to terms with their addiction to these foods, they will never lose their symptoms of intolerance or lose weight. Wendy, who we met on page 9, is a case of lifetime overweight who has benefited from the Food Addict's Diet.

Pubescent overweight ('puppy fat')
For boys this means that they were normal skinny lads until about the age of nine, when they began to gain weight, and possibly to this day they have never really lost it. For girls this happens a little later: the 'puppy fat' and the extra weight arrives at the age of about twelve,

and persists at least until the age of about sixteen, sometimes continuing into the twenties, or even longer.

There seem to be two factors at work here: it is well known that hormone changes at puberty create a prevailing feeling of lassitude and slight depression, and it is my belief that the child turns to food in search of a 'lift'. If particular foods, such as toast and sugary spreads, are found to be energising, then the child will opt for them continually, eventually becoming hooked on them. The extra calories they bring into the diet puts the weight on.

I am a good example of this kind of overweight: I was totally lacking in energy from the age of about nine, and used high-calorie foods such as glucose tablets in a desperate attempt to keep up with my energetic friends. Very soon I was basing my whole diet upon bread, sugar and cheese, eating constantly. I remained heavy for the rest of my life except when I was on a diet, which was more often than not. Only recently did I discover that only a few specific foods lay behind my weight problem, and not my lack of will power.

This kind of weight is the easiest to lose: the success stories from the slimming clubs are usually women in their twenties who were tubby in their teens and wanted to become slim. However, they are unlikely to keep the weight off, as we already know, because the food addictions that created the overweight are still at work.

Adult onset

Although slim until their twenties or even thirties, these people start to gain weight because of some event in their adult life. For men, this seems to be related to changes in lifestyle: a change to an easy life with access to lots of free food during the ubiquitous business lunch is enough to put weight on to the slimmest person unless he is very health conscious.

For women, the weight gain almost always has something to do with hormone changes. We have already mentioned puberty, but there are other changes, such as pregnancy or miscarriage, using the contraceptive pill, and of course the menopause and the 'middle-aged spread' that it brings.

The menopause seems to lower your metabolism, and the same diet that has kept you slim for years now begins to put weight on you for no apparent reason. I have successfully helped women who have gained weight for the first time during the menopause with the Food Addict's Diet. If we treat the problem as a manifestation of food intolerance we can see good results. The grain-free slimming option (for details, see page 144) has been particularly helpful for this group.

NEW HOPE

I hope in this chapter I have given you a few glimpses of what good health could mean to you – abounding energy and a joyful feeling of well-being, and an end to those annoying symptoms that drag you down but never make you really ill.

Also, you should now have a clearer picture of your present state of health. Understanding why you feel the way you do is the beginning to your cure. If you have lost hope that you will ever lose weight or feel better, then think again! This diet could be the answer you have been looking for: a simple, easy way to create a healthy diet for yourself and help your body heal itself, bringing you a new figure, new energy and new hope, and all for the price of four zero foods.

CHAPTER 3
You and Your Food

This chapter will focus on the way you actually eat. The four zero experiment will create many subtle changes in your relationship with your food, but there are many changes you can make in this area even before you begin the diet, so start now!

HOW OFTEN DO YOU EAT?

(Choose one response and delete those that do not apply to you.)

I eat breakfast every day/some days/less than twice a week/rarely/not all.

I eat lunch every day/some days/less than twice a week/rarely/not at all.

I eat after my evening meal every day/some days/less than twice a week/rarely/not at all.

I eat snacks about. . . .times a day.

My usual snack foods are:

....
....
....

In Chapter 7 you will be asked these questions again, to see if your eating habits have changed after trying the experiment.

A WEEK OF BIGGER BREAKFASTS

Breakfast, the most commonly skipped meal, is crucial to your health and energy. If you cannot face breakfast, at least introduce some kind of healthy food into your life before 10 o'clock each morning. If you eat very little breakfast or none at all, then you will not have as much energy as people who do – they can keep going through lunchtime and still have energy to spare at 4 o'clock. So, if you run out of energy by 11.30 a.m., try a week of bigger breakfasts, and see what happens to your energy, almost at once!

Paul and bigger breakfasts

Paul tried eating bigger breakfasts, and made money by it! He is a self-employed single man working with heavy cleaning machinery, and he has to cook his own meal at night. He normally relies on fast-cook food and uses alcohol for a quick energy boost in the evening. After doing some work for me he stood swaying with fatigue by 2.30 p.m., having spent five hours hard at work. All he had eaten that day was a bowl of cornflakes at 7 a.m., and he just wanted to go home and sit down.

I suggested that he would have more energy if he ate more often, and he might even make more money if he had the strength to fit other jobs into his day. So, just as an experiment, he tried two weeks of bigger breakfasts to see what happened to his energy.

Three weeks later he wrote to me, and reported a great increase in energy. He was taking on more work and finishing jobs a little sooner. He felt much happier, and his friends had already noticed his extra energy. Men like Paul who are self-employed must think of their health and energy as their principal asset, and a good breakfast is the key to that energy.

LUNCH

I believe that a good light lunch should be made up of three kinds of food: a small amount of a protein food such as meat, fish, nuts or seeds; plenty of fresh raw food such as fruit or a salad; and some energy food, such as bread, crackers or cakes. This is the kind of lunch you will eat on the Food Addict's Diet.

Fast-food lunches – usually based on the four zeros – are easy to buy and require no planning or forethought. By banning the four zeros, the Food Addict's Diet will make you take another look at lunch. If you miss lunch – especially after missing breakfast too – then you cannot expect to have much energy, or to keep good control over your appetite during the evening when you do finally have time to eat.

EVENING MEAL

During the trials for the Food Addict's Diet, I found that after the experiment 54 per cent of those questioned ate after their evening meal less often than before. This means that those long hungry evenings you remember from your last slimming diet will not feature this time, for it seems that on this diet you will feel quite satisfied after your evening meal. In fact, it was a common complaint on the trials that, in the early days of the experiment, they felt too full in the evening!

SNACKS

We do not eat often enough. Like our ape ancestors, we were designed to snack often rather than take one large meal in a day. Eating many times a day helps to keep up blood sugar, and will prevent you from getting so hungry that you forget your slimming intentions altogether!

As you will see when we come to the experiment, an important rule on the plan is to eat three times a day, and to eat snacks whenever you need them.

HOW FAST DO YOU EAT?

(Choose one and delete those that do not apply to you.)
   I eat: very quickly/quite quickly/at a normal speed/
quite slowly/very slowly.

Many people, especially the overweight, eat too
quickly. Even before you begin the diet, notice how fast
you eat, and *slow down*. Part of the joy of eating is to
savour your food, and you can't do that if you bolt it.
   Before you begin a meal, allow a few moments of
anticipation, when the saliva will begin to flow. When
you chew, let this saliva coat your food, savouring the
taste. See how long you can keep the food in your mouth
before you swallow. Never forget that chewing is the
principal pleasure of eating, so make the most of it!

DRINKING

Every day of your life your body needs about 1½ litres of
water to function normally. You can obtain some of this
water indirectly from the food you eat, but you should
also drink at least 1 litre of fluid a day. When you try the
four zero experiment, you will be expected to drink this
amount as part of your change in diet.

How much do you drink?
Choose one day to record your drinks.
   On this day I drank:
      ... glasses of water
      ... cups/mugs of tea
      ... cups/mugs of coffee
      ... glasses of fruit juice
      ... other drinks, including alcohol
....
This makes a total of ... litres of fluid.

NOTE: 1 litre is about 2 pint glasses/4 large mugs/5 small
mugs/6 glasses/7 cups.

There is a great deal you can do right now to increase your fluid consumption. We drink too little plain water, but when you hear what is in it, that is hardly surprising! Invest in a water filter, or try mineral waters. Just drinking extra tea and coffee will not improve your fluid balance very much, because coffee and tea increase urine production.

If you tend to eat hasty grills dressed with concentrated sauces, you will take very little fluid with your food, so you could think about eating more casseroles, stews and soups, because they can be a good source of extra fluid. Vegetables and fruit contain water, so eat them raw for their juice.

FLUID AND HEALTH

If you persistently drink less than your body needs, this can be very bad for you. I discovered how important drinking can be when I met Rachel, who was afraid to drink!

Rachel learns to drink

Rachel came forward to try the diet because she was five stones overweight. She suffered from chronic water retention and was generally feeling clogged up and run down. When I saw her normal food and drink chart it became clear that she hardly ever drank: two cups of tea a day was usually all she had. She had discovered that as she retained fluid her drinks made her heavier still, and so she had virtually stopped drinking in order to avoid putting on any extra pounds.

It was clear that the fluid question had to be tackled before Rachel began the diet. I warned her that she was risking kidney problems if she did not drink more, and she responded by increasing her intake of fluids, particularly as diluted fruit juices or soup.

She temporarily gained ten pounds in weight because she retained the fluid at first, but her urine output gradually increased from the usual trickle to a healthy flow with the help of the extra fluid. As the urine output increased so did her positive mood, and as she lost the extra fluid her weight gradually returned to its previous level.

Meanwhile, the muzzy feeling in her head cleared and her headaches, backache and chronic constipation eased. Then at last she began occasionally to experience a true feeling of thirst. This meant that she no longer had to remind herself to drink, which I took to mean that she was back to normal. Then we both agreed that she was ready to begin the diet, and she is now losing weight and no longer afraid of drinking.

ALCOHOL

The Food Addict's Diet is unusual as a slimming diet in that it does allow you to drink alcohol, but you will be asked to take a very careful look at the ingredients of the drinks you choose. On this diet you will only be allowed to take alcoholic drinks made from apples or grapes.

How many units do you drink in a week?
One unit of alcohol can be found in one half-pint of beer, one glass of table wine, one glass of sherry or port, or one small tot of spirits.

You can use this chart to record your alcohol consumption over the last seven days:

Sunday . . . . . units
Monday . . . . . units
Tuesday . . . . . units
Wednesday . . . . . units
Thursday . . . . . units
Friday . . . . . units
Saturday . . . . . units
Total units taken last week: . . . . . units

A sensible weekly limit is twenty-one units for men, and fourteen for women. If you are a man taking more than sixty units a week, or a woman taking more than forty units in a week, then you are endangering your health.[1] Alcohol is a poison, and overdoses can kill.

Addiction to alcohol

Even if you think you may be dependent on alcohol, this does not make you an 'alcoholic'. Addictions always operate along a sliding scale, and at their starting point they are barely noticeable. Facing up to a developing dependency can help you to prevent an addiction arising, so if you believe you may have a problem with alcohol it may help you to give some thought now to your present relationship with it.

Meanwhile, you will be able to continue enjoying alcoholic drinks while you are on the Food Addict's Diet. I will give you details of exactly which drinks you are allowed on page 117, which lists the foods you will be allowed to eat while on the diet.

SALT

Salt is sodium chloride, and we all need some in our diet; however, we tend to consume too much. Salt is added to many of our foods during processing or cooking, and it is not necessary to add any more at the table. It is an important source of sodium, but taking too much depletes the body of potassium. Sodium and potassium balance each other out in your body, so an excess or shortage of either of them can cause problems, particularly high blood pressure and oedema (swollen limbs, face, etc.).

SEARCH OUT SODIUM

Sodium is found in a wide range of food additives as well as salt, so if you eat a lot of packaged and processed foods – especially canned or dried – you are probably already consuming too much. Many processed foods are banned on the Food Addict's Diet, but you will notice that salt has already been added to some of the allowed foods, such as processed meats, so keep your consumption of these to a minimum. Always be aware of the salt and other forms of sodium that have been added to packeted food by reading the labels.

ARE YOU A SALT ADDICT?

If you are in the habit of shaking salt over every meal, stop it! Some people become addicted to salt, and find it very hard to give up. If you cannot imagine life without a shake of salt, then start reducing your intake right now, particularly if you have been told by your doctor to follow a low-sodium diet.

Notice how much salt you take in a day, and start to try and live without it. If your food tastes bland at first, sample some of the other spices and herbs, particularly garlic. In time you will begin to appreciate the subtle flavours in your food that were once masked by adding salt.

FATS

It appears that some of us have been led to believe that all fats and oils are a 'bad thing' for the health. This is largely true, but only where one particular kind of fat is taken to excess over another. Your good health relies not only on keeping your intake of fats and oils to a reasonable level, but also upon a good balance of saturated and unsaturated fat being available from your food.

A SIMPLE RULE

The existence of several kinds of fat was found to be one of the most confusing ideas in nutrition by some of my trials' candidates, who had decided to ignore the advice as they simply didn't understand it. I therefore translated the advice into a simple rule for them: avoid dairy products first, as this cuts out a major source of saturated fat; secondly, take all your other fats in a wide variety of ways and in as natural a form as possible. This means to eat the fat in meat as it occurs without overdoing it, but use oil too, and make sure that it is a cold-pressed oil that has not been refined or heated.

ESSENTIAL FATTY ACIDS

There has been much research recently into the effects on our health of the various fatty acids that make up the fats and oils we eat. Some are absolutely essential to good health, and are known as essential fatty acids, or EFAs. Unfortunately, they are easily destroyed or altered by heat or chemicals.

If you use a cold-pressed oil, you are getting natural, untouched EFAs. The only cold-pressed oil that is easy to come by in Britain is the greenish extra virgin olive oil that comes from Italy. There are others, but they are very expensive indeed. The other cheaper oils we normally use (corn, sunflower, or soya oil) have usually been chemically refined, so there is a risk that the EFAs in them have been damaged by processing.

You can read more about EFAs in Donald Rudin's book *The Omega Factor* (Sidgwick & Jackson, 1988).

MARGARINE AND HYDROGENATED FATS

To solidify oils and make them spreadable like butter, they are subjected to a chemical process called hydrogenation, which changes the fatty acids into a different form. On the Food Addict's Diet you will be allowed to use milk-free margarine as a substitute, but always remember that margarine is an entirely artificial food. Try to keep your consumption of margarine, and refined oils generally, to a minimum.

DON'T FORGET YOUR OILS!

When we come to Chapter 7 and you try the four zero experiment, I will repeatedly remind you to use olive oil. This is because essential fatty acids are needed every day, even when you are slimming. If you still prefer not to use oil, you can always take your EFAs by eating deep-sea fish, oily seeds and nuts. The chart on page 99 in Chapter 6 will help you to buy foods that are high in EFAs.

A LOOK AT YOUR PERSONAL DIET

Your personal diet is what you actually eat, not the family diet. Each individual member of your family eats a different diet, because there is always choice, and appetites vary enormously.

HOW HEALTHY IS YOUR PERSONAL DIET?

Underline the phrase that best describes your personal diet:
My personal diet is: always unhealthy/sometimes unhealthy/reasonably healthy/quite healthy/healthy/very healthy.

You will be asked this question again in Chapter 7 after the experiment: you may see some changes in how you answer this question!

However healthy you may *think* your diet to be at the moment, during the experiment you will find out what a truly varied and healthy diet can be.

However, if you find that your diet *is* healthy, and yet you are overweight or constantly troubled with minor ailments, what can you do? In that case you will need to look carefully at the actual foods you are eating and try the experiment to find the cause of the trouble. The foods you are allowed on the Food Addict's Diet will be as healthy as anything you are eating at the moment, so you will have nothing to lose by making the change, but everything to gain.

HOW DO YOU KNOW YOU ARE EATING HEALTHY FOOD?

We have already discussed the NACNE report, which uses words like 'saturated fat' or 'complex carbohydrates', but how does all this science relate to the foods you buy in the shop and the meals you serve your family? Now here is a simple way to define healthy food: it should be *real, whole, live and fresh*.

Real food

More than 70 per cent of what we spend on food goes on the processed variety. This kind of food no longer resembles the original food ingredients as they were found in nature, and it contains both natural and artificial food additives. There are many books about food additives and their effects.[2] Choose products that say 'no artificial ingredients' and at least you will not be buying chemicals to eat.

Eat your food raw whenever you can. There is a whole science devoted to using raw food as a healing diet.[3] The water contained in plants and vegetables is pure, and rich in those elusive trace elements, and the action of chewing and digesting raw foods encourages good digestion.

Whole food

Try to discover what the original natural form of your food is, by learning more about the food you eat. Then try to eat it in its whole form: for instance, try eating sunflower seeds instead of the oil, or the whole pineapple instead of its juice. Try wholegrains rather than flours; eat the whole animal, rather than just muscle meat; and eat whole fishes, bones included. When you eat fruit and vegetables, use them whole where you can: don't mash them to a pulp and destroy them.

Live food
It is important to realise that all food is alive until you harvest it or kill it. In living food, the vitamins and minerals are present in their natural state and combinations, the cell structures of each plant or animal are intact, so the little chemical messengers or enzymes are still there untouched. The water held in the tissues, rich in trace elements, is there untouched and absolutely fresh.

We should try to eat freshly picked or freshly killed food whenever possible to benefit from all this goodness.

Fresh food
All food processing is to do with preserving food and making it palatable for us to eat months after it would have rotted if left untreated. In fact, much of our food is many days old when we get it; some of it is artificially sweetened, preserved and flavoured; it has often been taken apart and reassembled in another form and, by the time we have finished freezing, boiling, drying, canning and irradiating the rest of it, it is well and truly dead.

TIME AND TROUBLE

It is so easy to say 'I haven't got time' to think about food, and we all do it. In order to follow the Food Addict's Diet, lose weight and feel better, you will have to think much more carefully about what you eat, at least at first.

Once you grasp the importance of taking care over what you eat, you will find that you do not begrudge the time. You will find that the rewards of the Food Addict's Diet will more than make up for any extra time you have to spend shopping or cooking. This is what Sarah discovered when she applied to try the diet.

Sarah thinks more about her food

When I suggested to Sarah, a friend of mine, that she should try the diet, she threw a dozen difficulties in the way: she leaves early in the morning to work, travels back late at night – sometimes about ten o'clock – and usually eats out in restaurants or cafes. She is constantly under stress, and needs quick and easy-to-prepare meals to keep her going. She has no time in the morning for breakfast, and when I suggested that she should take an early evening snack before returning home, she said there was nowhere suitable within easy reach of her work to do this. I suggested taking a packed lunch, but she enjoys eating out at lunchtime, as it helps her to relax. I suggested buying more fruit and vegetables and she said that she had no time to shop for them. She was resisting any attempt whatsoever to make a change in her diet, as she naturally resented having to make any diet change that would create any inconvenience or require extra time.

Four months later, as her job became more stressful, Sarah finally agreed to try the diet. Using all the initiative and drive that she put into her job, Sarah adopted the four zero plan fully and sensibly, and was surprised to find how easy it was. She found that she could after all find time for a good breakfast, and she saved time by preparing soups and casseroles the night before. She filled her freezer with pâtés, fish dishes and frozen vegetables for instant meals.

She discovered an Indonesian restaurant five minutes' walk from her workplace with a delightful chef who plied her with a variety of dishes allowed on the diet. When entertaining a customer at a French restaurant, she found items on the menu that obeyed the rules, and sipped a glass of white wine.

On her initiative, a small microwave cooker was installed at work in the kitchen alongside the kettle, and hot soup is now served as often as tea. Sarah has encouraged two other girls to join her, and they have found a cafe open in the evenings that will provide just a bowl of soup. Before returning home at night, they come in for their soup and return home refreshed.

The four zero plan has opened up new ways of eating, rekindled an interest in cooking, and it has helped Sarah to see how her feelings of stress arise directly out of her diet.

THE PRICE OF HEALTHY EATING

How expensive is the Food Addict's Diet? When you start to base your diet on more whole, fresh basic ingredients, will you be able to afford it?

Buying convenience food saves time, but also costs money: this kind of food is always more expensive than buying basic food ingredients. For instance, a can of vegetable soup costs very much more than the small quantity of vegetables you would need to make the same amount for yourself. The extra cost is the price of convenience.

Buying fresh foods costs less money but takes more time: you must shop for them at least twice a week, for fresh fruits and vegetables do not keep a whole week, even in the fridge. So many processed foods contain the four zeros that you will buy more fresh foods and basic ingredients when you are on the Food Addict's Diet. Fresh foods are much cheaper than processed foods, and you will be surprised at how well you can eat while spending no more money than before.

COOKING WITH CARE

The Food Addict's Diet will force you to cook more foods for yourself, simply because very few of the allowed ingredients are available in handy packaged form.

Cooking for health is becoming a lost art. Our too-heavy reliance on processed food and pre-packed meals has increased our dependence upon the four zeros, and I believe that this overdependence is the main reason for our unhealthy British diet. There is a solution to this problem, and it lies in your kitchen: cook for health, not convenience.

So, if you must cook your vegetables, keep the precious juices carefully and add them to soups and casseroles. We British boil our vegetables to a mush in the name of good digestion.

PREPARING FOR THE PLAN

The ideas I have given you in this chapter can be brought into action at once, and I hope you will never forget them. You should now know how important food is: how carefully you must shop for it, and even how well you must chew it! You also should realise the importance of having plenty of fluids to drink, and eating three good meals a day.

If you put these ideas into action straightaway, then by the time you are ready to begin the four zero experiment you will have already taken an important step in your journey to better health.

CHAPTER 4
Making a Food Diary

Here is where the fun begins: you will now have a clearer idea of how healthy you really are, and what changes could be made in your eating and drinking habits even before you begin the diet. This chapter will give you a completely new angle on your food, and you will be able to use what you have learned to find out how varied your personal diet really is.

ANALYSING YOUR FOOD

When you start hunting through your daily diet looking for zero foods in disguise, you will need to take a close look at the basic ingredients that were used to make your food. You will have to see bread as wheat flour, yeast, salt and water; butter as a form of cows' milk; plain chocolate as sugar and cocoa, and so on. Anyone who enjoys cooking with basic ingredients will find this easy, but if you eat much of your food in pre-packaged form, some of the ingredients you discover when you read the labels may take you by surprise!

To be successful on the Food Addict's Diet, this new way of looking at foods must become second nature. We will start with a three-day food diary made now, before you start the diet, and use this to make comparisons later. To make your food diary I want you to record everything you eat and drink over three consecutive days, to analyse it and record which basic food ingredients were used to make it. You will find a form on page 75 to record the information.

FINDING THE BASIC INGREDIENTS

Analysing your food in this way can be very interesting indeed! You probably already know the basic ingredients of some of the foods you eat, but if you don't, then consult your recipe books. You may find you are eating zero foods in disguise, such as butter used as an ingredient in biscuits. In that case, note the original basic food, not the disguise. The butter in the biscuit will be noted as 'cows' milk', for that is where the butter originally came from. Do the same for Oxo stock (beef) and pastry (milk, wheat), and so on.

Some of the ingredients, such as flavouring and caffeine drinks, are not classed as food. These have no food value, and they can be marked 'NFV'.

Some processed foods have a series of unknown and mysterious ingredients in them, and so are difficult to analyse. As so many of them contain the four zeros, and thus are banned on the diet, there will only be a few left to decipher. Meanwhile, you can list stock cubes simply as: 'stock cube', and margarine as: 'oils – various'. For any others, read the labels and just list the main food ingredients.

In Chapter 7 you will be given a chance to repeat this exercise while you are on the Food Addict's Diet, and then you will see clearly the changes the diet has made in the way you eat.

To help you to make your own food diary, I have analysed one day's diet, which was supplied by one of my trials candidates, Deborah, as her diet record before starting the experiment.

Deborah's diet analysed

Breakfast	*ingredients*
Weetabix	wheat

71

milk	cows' milk
sugar	sugar
two slices of toast	wheat
	yeast
	salt (NFV)
margarine	oils, various
marmalade	orange
	sugar
tea	tea (NFV)
milk	cows' milk
glass of orange juice	orange

Mid-morning snack

coffee	coffee (NFV)
milk	cows' milk
two ginger biscuits	wheat
	sugar
	cows' milk (butter)
	ginger (NFV)

Lunch

hamburger	beef
	onion flavouring (NFV)
roll	wheat
	yeast
onions	onion
lettuce	lettuce
chips	potato
	vegetable oil
Coca-Cola	sugar

Mid-afternoon snack

tea	tea (NFV)
milk	cows' milk
malted milk biscuits	wheat
	barley
	cows' milk
	sugar

Teatime snack

tea	tea (NFV)
packet of crisps	potato
	vegetable oil
	salt (NFV)

Evening meal

chicken and leek casserole	chicken
	onion
	tomato
	leeks
	stock cubes
broccoli	broccoli
mashed potato	potato
banana	banana
slice of fruit cake	wheat
	cows' milk (butter)
	sugar
	grapes (raisins)
	grapes (sultanas)
	cherry (glacé)
	almonds
	eggs
coffee	coffee (NFV)
milk	cows' milk

Making a list of ingredients

Now we have discovered what exactly has been eaten, it is time to make a list of the ingredients used to arrive at a daily total. To do this, list each food under the correct heading.

Ingredients from Deborah's diet

meat:	beef
	chicken
fish:	none
eggs:	chicken's egg (in cake)

73

beans and pulses:	none
seeds:	none
nuts:	almonds (in cake)
fruit:	orange (juice)
	banana
	grapes (raisins)
	grapes (sultanas)
	cherries (glacé)
vegetables:	onion
	lettuce
	tomato
	leeks
	potato
	vegetable oils in margarine, chips and crisps
grains and starch foods:	wheat (flour)
sugars:	sugar
milks:	cows' milk
other foods:	yeast (in bread)
	stock cube
no food value (NFV):	onion flavouring
	salt
	Coca-Cola
	tea
	coffee

There are twenty foods on this list. (I have not counted the NFV ingredients. Also, I have counted both stock cubes and the oils in margarine and in crisps and chips as single foods, because it is very difficult to find out exactly what ingredients have been used.)

YOUR PERSONAL FOOD DIARY

Make a full list of *absolutely all food and drink* consumed
by you over three consecutive days. Make a list under the
word 'ingredients' of the basic ingredients of the dishes
you choose. Laid out below is a form for Day One. Photocopy or copy it by hand for Days Two and Three.

Day one (Date ....)

Before rising   *ingredients*

....
....
....

Breakfast

....
....
....
....
....
....
....
....

Mid-morning snack

....
....
....
....
....
....

Lunch

....
....
....
....
....
....
....

. . . .
. . . .

Mid-afternoon snack

. . . .
. . . .
. . . .
. . . .
. . . .
. . . .

Teatime snack

. . . .
. . . .
. . . .
. . . .
. . . .
. . . .

Evening meal

. . . .
. . . .
. . . .
. . . .
. . . .
. . . .
. . . .
. . . .
. . . .
. . . .
. . . .

Before bed

. . . .
. . . .
. . . .

During the night

. . . .
. . . .
. . . .

A TRULY VARIED DIET

If we were to make a list of all the various foods eaten in Britain in, say, the eighteenth century, it would be very long indeed, and would include all kinds of wild herbs, vegetables and fruits, together with some animals and birds we would never think of eating today. At that time a much larger proportion of people lived off the land, and took more advantage of free, wild foods than we do today. Now that so many of us live in towns and cities this has changed: we now eat only what we can buy.

How long would that list of foods be now? On page 98 you can find out: there you will find a comprehensive list of the foods available for you to eat at some time during the year here in Britain. There are more than 200 foods on this list, but it is still a lot shorter than it would have been two centuries ago. Our modern attitude to food makes it shorter still, for most of us seem to be afraid to experiment with less usual ingredients. Today we build our daily diet from a small group of about fifty foods. We have become dependent on them, and many of us are well on the way to becoming addicted to some of them.

DEPENDENCE ON OUR STAPLES

If you take another look at Deborah's diet on pages 71–4 you may notice how many times she ate the four zero foods that day. In a single day she ate wheat 6 times, milk 8 times, potatoes 3 times and sugar 6 times, even though she adds no sugar to her drinks.

Like Deborah, we have all built our seemingly 'varied' diet upon a small group of foods served in many different ways. For instance, the four main ingredients of her hamburger lunch (beef, wheat, onion and lettuce) could reappear in several other disguises, such as a beef salad with a bread roll and pickled onion; part of the ingredients needed for a spaghetti bolognese; or a steak and onion pie to go with chips and salad.

Now you can see that this so-called 'variety' is a myth,

77

perpetuated by the imaginations of our cooks and the marketing genius of our food-processing industry. It is true that some of us do try to make use of less usual ingredients, but even so we are not making full use of all the 200 foods available for us to buy. We should – for variety is not just more interesting, but essential for good health.

VARIETY AND GOOD HEALTH

There are about forty essential nutrients that cannot be manufactured in the body, or cannot be made fast enough for the body's needs. This means that at least some part of the supply must come from the diet.

These are:

9 amino acids: histidine, leucine, iso-leucine, lysine, methionine, phenylalanine, threonine, tryptophan and valine.

13 vitamins: retinol (Vitamin A), thiamine (Vitamin B1), riboflavin (Vitamin B2), niacin (Vitamin B3), pantothenic acid (Vitamin B5), pyridoxine (Vitamin B6), folic acid (Vitamin B9), cobalamin (Vitamin B12), biotin, PABA (para-aminobenzoic acid), ascorbate (Vitamin C), tocopherol (Vitamin E), Vitamin K.

15 minerals: sodium, potassium, calcium, magnesium, phosphorus, iron, zinc, copper, manganese, chromium, selenium, molybdenum, chlorine, fluoride, iodine.

other: water, fibre and energy.

(*Source*: Xandria Williams, *What's in My Food?* (Prism Press, Australia, 1988.)

If you want to know which are the best sources of each of these nutrients, and how much you need of each for good health, read Earl Mindell's *The Vitamin Bible* (Arlington Books, 1979; reprinted 1987).

It would take more than a single day's food to obtain enough of all forty essential nutrients for good health, even though some are only needed in minute amounts. The important thing to bear in mind therefore is not just your daily diet, but which foods you eat over a period of several days, or even weeks.

Apart from these forty essential nutrients, there are twenty or more other nutrients that can be made in your body, but can also be obtained directly from your diet. If you only eat a limited number of foods you run the risk of becoming deficient in one or other of these 60 nutrients. This can make you feel run down, and could explain some of the symptoms we discussed in Chapter 2. There is no small group of foods that will give us all the nutrients we need: your diet must be based on a wide variety of ingredients if you want to be healthy.

MAKING A THREE-DAY VARIETY SCORE

To make a truly varied diet for yourself you will need to take a longer-term look at what you eat, and think more carefully about your choice of food – not just every day, but over the weeks and months. Perhaps you could aim to have tasted every food on the list of 200 by the end of the year.

Another way to increase variety is to use a variety scoring system. This system would have to include foods eaten over at least three days. I found with the help of some of my diet trials candidates that it is possible to use about fifty ingredients in three days, so I decided that fifty should be the optimum score.

This is the scoring system we developed:

    10–20   dangerously monotonous
    20–25   rather boring and repetitive
    25–35   healthy average
    35–40   very healthy, varied diet
    40 +   excellent!

YOUR PERSONAL VARIETY SCORE

Now that you have a food diary with details of all the various ingredients you have eaten over three days, you can make a three-day variety score for your own personal diet.

To do this, simply list on a piece of paper the different ingredients you wrote in your food diary during all three days (as we did for Deborah's one-day diet on pages 71-4), making sure to list each ingredient only once – and beware of disguises!

Now add up all the ingredients you listed, and note the total below:

In the three days I ate . . . . . ingredients.

This is your personal three-day variety score. How does it compare with the table above? In Chapter 7 you will be able to find out your score when you are on the Food Addict's Diet – you may be surprised at what you discover!

HOW VARIED IS YOUR DIET?

You may have discovered through this exercise that your diet is not as varied as it could be. If so, it cannot be described as 'balanced' either, because it is based on too few ingredients to be so. During the trials we found that as variety increases, the diet does become healthier in many other ways. The diet trials also highlighted an important fact: one of the insidious effects of food addiction is that it swamps your normal instincts for food choice.

You have an inbuilt 'instinct' for seeking out the right food to meet your body's needs; this has guided hunter-gatherers through many hundreds of generations. This 'guide' is alive and well, and waiting within us to be allowed to function, as you will soon discover – once your addiction has been cured!

CHAPTER 5
Are You A Food Addict?

In this chapter we will look at the problem that lies at the core of this book: your personal relationship with your food. We will learn more about addiction itself, and discover the very essence of pleasure. We will look at some of the reasons why we become addicted, and learn how we can take the same eight steps to overcome any kind of addiction. We will speculate about how it might feel to live without the four zero foods for a while, and finally we will look at the role of hunger in food addiction and food choices.

WHY DO WE BECOME ADDICTED?

There are two possible explanations for addictive cravings, and they both have a part to play in food addiction.

ENDORPHINS

Stress lies at the very root of many kinds of addiction, for if you are an addict it is not the 'fix' itself you are addicted to, but the effect of endorphins. These are hormone-like chemicals that kill pain in much the same way as morphine and also bring a feeling of pleasure and satisfaction.

When you are under stress the stress hormone

adrenaline is produced. This quickens all your bodily pro-
cesses and sharpens your perception, and at the same time
endorphins are produced in your brain. This is why most
of us find some stress thrilling and enjoyable, for it is
our endorphins that create this enjoyment. We can even
become addicted to stress itself, just because we like the
feeling it brings.

Some of our foods contain drug-like chemicals that
imitate the effects of endorphins. I believe that this is
why we become addicted to the solanine in potatoes and
several other foods and drugs (see pages 159-74).

Dr John Brostoff, in his book *Food Allergy and Intolerance* (Bloomsbury, 1989), suggested yet another reason
for addictive cravings: when the proteins found in some
foods (including two of our zero foods – milk and wheat)
are digested using human enzymes under laboratory conditions, peptides are produced that are very similar to
endorphins. Dr Brostoff suggests that the sense of comfort and well-being that these foods produce in some
people could be due to the effects of these peptides derived
from food. This could well explain our addiction to wheat
and milk.

ADDICTION AND FOOD INTOLERANCE

People who are intolerant to a food react by producing
some kind of symptom after they eat it, such as you found
listed in Chapter 2 (page 41). They also usually show signs
of becoming addicted to it. This is so common that looking for addictions at work is a useful method of diag-
nosing food intolerance, as you can see on page 178.

There are various explanations of why people tend to
become hooked on the very food that makes them ill, but
the most usual explanation is to call this kind of addiction
'adaptation'.

The adaptation theory
This theory is based upon the observation that your body
is capable of becoming adapted to even the most uncom-

fortable situations, given enough time. If you happen to take regular overdoses of any food, your body will eventually adapt to having it around constantly in such large quantities. An overdose of food can be eaten all at once as a 'binge', or over many days and years as a diet based on a very limited number of foods. How well you manage to adapt depends on how much adjustment your body has to make to accommodate the overdose.

If you show intolerance symptoms whenever you eat a particular food, this means that you are having difficulty adapting to it. If you are young and healthy you can become so perfectly adapted to any diet, however narrow, that there is no sign of illness at all, even after constant overdoses. Only later, when your body gradually becomes less efficient at adapting, do signs of intolerance begin to show. Other people, though, show food intolerance symptoms throughout life, and they are usually members of 'atopic' families – that is, families with an inherited tendency to be bad at adaptation. In these families this manifests itself as a variety of food intolerances and allergic reactions, taking different forms among different members of the family.

Adaptation and addiction

Once your body has adapted, successfully or not, it seems to want to stay that way! If the food you have become adapted to is no longer present, your body begins almost at once to readjust. We call this 'withdrawal'. If you then take another dose your body will adapt once more and return to what has always felt 'normal' to you, but in fact is not normal at all! The urge to maintain the constant state of adaptation is very strong indeed.

This is how, when we become adapted to overdoses of a food, we develop adaptive cravings for it. Cows' milk and sugar are given to some babies in the very earliest days of life, and wheat and potatoes not long after. Most of us have taken at least one of the four zero foods every day of our lives since then. It is small wonder then that

83

we find it hard to live without them, experience withdrawal symptoms when they are removed, and crave a further dose of them to put us back to 'normal'.

HOW ADDICTIONS DEVELOP

As a result of my personal observations of addicts of various kinds, I have noticed a definite series of stages that people go through as they gradually become addicted. To illustrate this clearly, I will use Tony as an example; Tony was addicted to cigarettes. Later we will meet Joan, whose addiction to food developed in just the same way as Tony's addiction to tobacco.

Tony's story
Stage 1: discovery
During a period of unhappiness, boredom, frustration or stress, our potential addict discovers a 'fix' that will bring relief from stress, a feeling of satisfaction, or a lift in mood. This could be anything: a piece of chocolate cake, a nice cup of tea, or a jog around the block. Tony discovered nicotine gave him a lift quite by chance when he was introduced to smoking by his friends.

Stage 2: increased consumption
As taking the fix feels good, the tendency is to use it more and more as time goes by. Tony began to smoke whenever he was under stress or in need of a 'lift'. His consumption quickly rose to over twenty cigarettes a day, and he began to spend more money and time on ensuring a regular supply of tobacco.

He increased his smoking still further when he got his first job, which was not a success, and he was very unhappy for the three months until he left. That period of stress seemed to 'set' his addiction to cigarettes, even though he then moved to another job where he was much happier.

Stage 3: an inability to stop

Even after making several firm and determined decisions to stop smoking, Tony found he could not. Again and again he failed in his resolution. Various psychological reasons have been put forward to explain why addictions are hard to break, but there is a purely physical reason that we should never ignore: addictive cravings.

This craving feeling comes whenever the fix has not been available for any length of time – from a few minutes to a few days. Addictive cravings are an over-whelming desire to take more of the fix as soon as possible. If there is also a sudden increase in stress, the craving can increase enormously.

However, if the fix is withdrawn completely, the cravings do not go on increasing indefinitely, but die down after a few days, only returning whenever there is an increase in stress. In theory, the best way to beat addiction is to do it gradually, but in practice it never works, because cravings can be maintained by regular doses of the fix, however small. So even though Tony tried all kinds of methods to cut down the number of cigarettes he smoked, he was never successful until he gave up smoking entirely.

Stage 4: the addiction itself becomes a problem

Addictions have to be paid for, and they can affect health, work habits and relationships. Often the addict refuses to admit to the problem, because he has no wish to be thought weak.

When Tony's mother dared to suggest that he was addicted to cigarettes he became very angry. He became defiant, and claimed that he was 'entitled to at least one vice'. His health and work began to suffer as his anxiety about his addiction was added to the effects of the smoke on his health.

Joan's story

I hope by this story to show you that food addiction develops through four stages, in just the same way as any

85

other kind of addiction. Joan proved that she was an addict, and solved her problem with the Food Addict's Diet.

When I met her, Joan had a great attachment to starchy foods: bread, crackers, biscuits, cakes, crisps, pasta and pastry. She liked a sweet taste, and enjoyed sweets and chocolate, but given the choice, she always chose wheat or potato-based foods. She found that if she felt low and bored she got a satisfaction from a starchy meal that a low-starch 'slimming' meal did not seem to provide. As a result, she was two stones overweight (stage 1).

She ate what she felt was a normal, balanced diet, but she knew that some foods were 'naughty but nice'. She could resist cream cakes and ice cream, but she found jacket potatoes, toast and muesli irresistible. Her need for starchy food ruled her appetite, and as a result she found it hard to limit her calorie intake (stage 2).

If she began a slimming diet where starchy foods were restricted, after a while she craved them. The slightest amount of stress found her making excuses to have them. Her body would yearn for 'just a little', but a little would soon become a lot, and her diet would break down in an orgy of eating (stage 3).

She lacked confidence in herself as a result of this lack of control, and naturally felt depressed every time a diet failed in this way, which was at least once a month. She was so anxious not to face what seemed to her a terrible weakness, that she became angry and defensive if the subject of her excess weight was discussed. She had a hang-up about her body, hating its fatness and yet longing to love it as it was: she had considered trying psychotherapy for this problem. For twenty-six years Joan had been dieting, and had broken slimming diets hundreds of times. The toll on her self-confidence of this catalogue of failures was enormous (stage 4).

You can see that the four stages in the development of Joan's addiction to food are as clear as in Tony's story, and you will be glad to know that both of them successfully brought their addictions under control by using the same methods.

EIGHT STEPS ON THE ROAD TO SUCCESS

By observing addicts of various kinds successfully bringing their consumption under control, I have created eight steps that need to be taken regardless of the kind of addiction. As Tony and Joan overcame their addictions, they both went through the same stages:

1. Admission and awareness
Know the effects of the fix on your mind and body and find a reason for giving it up.

Tony watched a documentary on television and was horrified at the things that tobacco can do. He decided that he should give up smoking. Joan had read quite a lot about food and health, and knew that she tended to overeat and should therefore cut her food consumption.

2. Giving up
Just make a start and survive the first few days.

Tony knew that he could not reduce his consumption gradually, because he had tried before. The only answer was to cut out cigarettes completely, so he did. Joan agreed to try the Food Addict's Diet and give up milk, sugar, wheat and potatoes completely, and she made a start on the following Monday.

3. See an end to cravings
Notice your cravings begin to die away after the first five days.

In the first few days without tobacco Tony had to cope with strong cravings for it. The first four days were the worst, after which he actually forgot about cigarettes for short periods of the day! Going into places where he usually smoked reawakened the craving, so he avoided

87

pubs, clubs and friends who smoked for the first few weeks.

On the fifth day on the diet Joan awoke feeling fine. She hardly thought about toast or potatoes that day. The next day she actually forgot to eat lunch until 2.30 p.m., something that had never happened to her before.

4. Gain rewards

Begin to see the advantages of giving up, and use them to keep you going.

Tony felt better, calmer, and had stopped coughing. He noticed the stale smell of tobacco more and became very sensitive to it, finding it sickly and unpleasant. His food tasted better, he had more energy, felt more alive, and took pleasure in new things.

Joan found that she could eat more often without guilt. Food tasted really good, and for once she knew when to stop, as she felt really full up after her meals. She felt livelier, happier and slimmer than she had felt for years, and lost five pounds in the first three weeks.

5. Feeling deprived

Be aware that a sense of deprivation will set in eventually, either within days or weeks.

For Tony, a sense of deprivation set in after a few weeks, when he just couldn't face the idea of the rest of his life without a fix from tobacco.

After the second weekend, Joan felt as if she had been on the diet for ever.

6. Lapse and collapse

Be prepared to break down many times and know how to make a new start.

After a quarrel with his girlfriend, Tony went out with his pals to the pub and had a cigarette. The next day he smoked five, the next, ten.

Joan made a fruit cake and ate some, and the next day there was some left over and she could not resist it. Where had all that will power gone?

7. *A feeling of control*
Feel your confidence in your control growing every month until small lapses no longer matter.

Eventually Tony managed to cope with those first four days without smoking, and get to stage 3 where his cravings died. He had at last discovered what he had to do to stay off cigarettes.

Joan breaks her diet about every four or five weeks, just for a day or two, but she now knows that wheat has a hold over her, and she always avoids it where possible to stay in control.

8. *Acceptance*
Face the fact that addiction is for life, and that the intake of your fix must always be carefully controlled.

Tony is careful not to think that he is really over smoking. He knows that he will be cured the day he can take just one cigarette and stop there, and he is not at that stage yet.

Joan knows that she will never be able to eat the way she did before without becoming addicted again. She is no longer a food addict, though, thanks to the Food Addict's Diet.

ARE YOU AN ADDICT?

How hard would it be for you to live entirely without each of the following basic ingredients in their various forms for just three weeks? (Circle the description that applies to you.)

Wheat	impossible/very hard/hard/easy/very easy.
Sugar	impossible/very hard/hard/easy/very easy.
Cows' milk	impossible/very hard/hard/easy/very easy.
Potatoes	impossible/very hard/hard/easy/very easy.

In Chapter 7 you will be asked these questions again. Then you may find a difference between how you now imagine it would be, and the reality. Our experience on the trials showed us that the effects of giving up the four zeros on the Food Addict's Diet can take anyone by surprise!

WHAT ARE YOUR FAVOURITES?

Which are your nine favourite dishes (e.g., shepherd's pie, roast beef and Yorkshire pudding, fruit cake, etc.)?

Write the name of each dish in the space provided, and then circle any of the four zero foods that have been used to make it.

I enjoy eating most:

Soups and starters   (Which zeros have been used?)
a .... wheat/milk/sugar/potato
b .... wheat/milk/sugar/potato

Savoury dishes
c .... wheat/milk/sugar/potato
d .... wheat/milk/sugar/potato
e .... wheat/milk/sugar/potato

Desserts
f .... wheat/milk/sugar/potato
g .... wheat/milk/sugar/potato

Teatime treats
h .... wheat/milk/sugar/potato
i .... wheat/milk/sugar/potato

I am prepared to hazard a guess that there are very few dishes mentioned above that do not contain at least one of the four zero foods! You will probably be surprised at how much you miss some of the zero foods on the experiment and how little you miss others.

ADDICTION AND HUNGER

Hunger is a very subtle force moulding our entire diet through our choice of food. Your natural hunger is stimulated or 'switched on' by shortage, and satisfied or 'switched off' by excess. On the other hand, your addictive cravings are unnatural, are switched on by your need for a fix, and have no built-in switch-off, so cannot be easily satisfied.

TRUE HUNGER

A few hours without food will usually create a feeling of 'true' hunger. A lack of food can cause weakness of the limbs, a dizzy feeling, or even faintness; but for some people it feels very good. In fact, it is possible to last a long time without food and feel no sensation of 'hunger' at all. The sight and smell of food sets your gastric juices going and this 'switches on' true hunger. The 'switch-off' for this hunger is just food – anything will do.

DEFICIENCY HUNGER

This hunger is switched on by a shortage of a particular nutrient in the diet. Your body can hold reserves of some vitamins and most minerals but, even so, supplies can run out and subtle shortages are developing all the time. Being able to provide for your body's deficiencies is very important for good health, and this is the purpose of deficiency hunger.

The switch-off for this kind of hunger is a supply of the nutrient currently in short supply. A vague feeling of unease can persist until the deficiency is satisfied.

BALANCE HUNGER

This kind of hunger is designed to prevent overdoses of food. The 'switch-on' is the desire for something a bit different to eat, such as a crisp salad after a stodgy meal. The 'switch-off' is any kind of excess⟩

ADDICTIVE CRAVINGS

You now know what addictive cravings are, but when you feel them at work they feel just like 'hunger'. They are the reason why you can still be 'hungry' when you know you have eaten enough. In this way, they interfere with your true hunger switch-off. They tend to drive you only towards a few favourite foods, so you neglect others, and create subtle deficiencies that you do not notice.

They are the reason why people, especially the overweight, find it hard to control their appetite, and they are the principal target of this book.

OVERCOME YOUR CRAVINGS FOR EVER WITH THE FOOD ADDICT'S DIET!

Natural hunger is a gentle affair and quite different from addictive cravings. Cravings stop you in your tracks and send you in search of refreshment at once, while your natural hunger is not so urgent. As soon as your natural hunger is back in charge during the experiment, you will only eat what you need when you need it. The Food Addict's Diet will replace the pleasure you once gained from your addiction to food with a wonderful feeling of well-being and vitality – one that will make you feel more alive than any fix could ever do.

At the start of this chapter you may have felt a little disturbed by the idea of food addiction as a feature of your life, but when you have rediscovered your natural hunger, your will power and your taste for real, whole, natural food, you will happily admit that it is true: you were once a food addict, but it's now in the past.

Part Two
The Four Zero
Experiment

CHAPTER 6
Foods You Can Eat

In this chapter I will introduce you to the 200 foods that you can eat on your new diet without the four zeros, and provide some menus to set you on your way. At the end of this chapter you can fill in a self-assessment questionnaire to record how you feel just before you begin the experiment, and use it later to make comparisons.

The prospect of living without the four zeros may seem rather bleak at the moment, but this chapter should prove to you how wrong you are. The Food Addict's Diet will be one of the most varied and interesting diet plans you have ever been offered.

SUBSTITUTES

As soon as you begin to live without your four favourites, you will initially find that no meal seems complete without them – or a close approximation to them – so here are details of the substitutes you can use.

SUBSTITUTES FOR WHEAT-BASED FOODS

You will think of your own ways of substituting other foods for wheat, but basically it means using all the other grains and starch foods.

Other grains used whole
Millet; rice; barley; buckwheat.

Other grains used as flakes
Rice; oats; millet; rye.

Other grains used as a meal or as flour
Barley meal or flour; buckwheat flour; cornflour; oatmeal; rice flour; rye flour.

Other starch foods
Sago; tapioca, arrowroot.

Starchy root vegetables
See Potato entry below.

Flour for baking
Cornflour; rye flour; soya flour (available from health-food shops); barley flour (available from some good health-food shops); fine ground oatmeal; gram flour (made from chick peas, available from health-food shops and some supermarkets).

Bread
100 per cent wholemeal rye crispbread (Ryvita, Finncrisp, Scanda Crisp, etc.); 100 per cent rye bread (available from good bakers); quick rice bread (see recipe, page 246); rice cakes; oatcakes (be sure they are sugar-free).

Make your own bread or rolls with non-wheat flours (see 'Flour' entry above).

Biscuits and cakes
Make your own with non-wheat flours (see recipes, pages 282–3).

Pasta
Buckwheat noodles (available from good health-food shops).

SUBSTITUTES FOR COWS' MILK

Liquid milk
Goats' milk; sheep's milk; soya milk (buy sugar-free from health-food shops); nut milks (see recipes, page 245).

Butter
Tomor margarine is milk-free. It can be bought from health-food shops and some supermarkets.

Cream
Soya dessert (Plamil sugar-free desserts, available from health-food shops); almond cream (see recipe, page 245).

Cheese
Goats' milk cheese (Fromage de chèvre); ewes' milk cheese (Roquefort).

Milk in your tea/coffee
Soya milk; goats' milk; sheep's milk.

Other hot drinks which taste good without milk
Earl Grey or jasmine tea, made fresh and not too strong; black coffee; various herb teas (available from health-food shops and some good supermarkets); hot diluted lemon juice sweetened with honey.

SUBSTITUTES FOR POTATOES

Whole boiled potatoes
Sweet potatoes; parsnips.

Mashed potato:
Swede; carrot; parsnip; turnip; sweet potato; pease pudding (see recipe, page 253); other beans cooked to a pulp.

Chips
Parsnip chips (see recipe, page 249); sweet potato chips (see recipe, page 248).

Roasted:
Sweet potatoes; parsnips.

Stew-strengtheners:
Grains and starch foods (see 'Wheat: Flour', entry above). Starchy root vegetables (see recipes, page 248): parsnips; turnips; swedes; sweet potatoes.

Pulses
Lentils; dried peas.

SUBSTITUTES FOR BEET AND CANE SUGAR

In your drinks
Honey; fructose (available from health-food shops and some good supermarkets); maple syrup.

Baking
Fructose; date purée (see recipe, page 248); dried fruits (prunes, figs, raisins, currants, sultanas, apricots, etc.).

Sweetening bitter fruit
Artificial sweeteners; maple syrup; fructose; apple juice concentrate (available from health-food shops); date purée (good with rhubarb; see recipe, page 282).

THE 200 FOODS

While you are avoiding the four zero foods, your new diet will be built from the 200 foods that are left, all of which you can eat with impunity. These fall into eight basic groups, and I have listed them below. There are some differences in availability of produce around the world, mainly among highly perishable foods such as fresh fish, fruit and vegetables. If you do not live in the United Kingdom, then adapt the table to suit yourself by crossing out any unobtainable foods and filling in any missing ones in the space provided.

ANIMAL PRODUCTS

Fish
(key: (E) = rich in essential fatty acids)

Freshwater fish
bream

salmon (E)

Other . . . .

trout (E)

Sea Fish
anchovy (E)

brill

cod and cod's roe

coley

eels

haddock and smoked
   haddock

hake

halibut

herring/kipper/bloater
   (E)

lemon sole

mackerel and smoked
   mackerel (E)

monkfish

pilchard (E)

plaice

red mullet

rock salmon

sardine (E)

sea bream

skate

sprats (E)

sturgeon (caviar) (E)

tuna

turbot

whitebait

whiting

Other . . . .

Shellfish
clam

cockles

crab

crayfish

lobster

mussels

Other . . . .

prawn/scampi

scallop

shrimp

whelks

winkles

NOTE: Fish is a very important source of calcium, especially those fish that have small edible bones that don't stick in the throat. Look at the Calci-Counter on page 286 and note which fish are rich sources of calcium. Some fish (marked (E) on the list) are good suppliers of some essential fatty acids, particularly those that live in cold, dark waters.

Meats

On the hoof
beef and veal   pork
goat   venison
lamb or mutton
Other . . . .

Game
grouse   pheasant
hare   pigeon
partridge   rabbit
Other . . . .

Other animals
snails
Other . . . .

Poultry
chicken   goose
duck   turkey
Other . . . .

NOTE: For prepared meats like haslet, faggot, haggis, etc., read the labels to find which animal the meat comes from. We eat many parts of the animal – the liver, the heart, the brains, etc. Remember that when you eat chicken liver, for example, you are still eating chicken, and when you eat tripe it is still beef.

Offal (that is all the bits that are not muscle meat) is rich in protein, with the added bonus of extra B vitamins and iron – and all at a much lower price than muscle meat. Avoid prepared meats such as sausages or ham as they often contain the banned ingredients, and in any case they are much more expensive than the equivalent weight of fresh meat.

Eggs

chickens' eggs	goose eggs
duck eggs	quails' eggs
Other eggs	

NOTE: Most people eat nothing but hens' eggs, so bring more variety into your diet by using goose, turkey and duck eggs in recipes for cakes and puddings, but do not eat them soft-boiled, or used for meringue, unless they are known to have been laid under strictly hygienic conditions.

Milks

ewes'/sheep's milk	goats' milk
Other animal milks	

NOTE: These other animal milks have been suggested as a substitute for cows' milk, but try the various nut and seed milk substitutes instead (see page 245): you may be surprised at how cheap and delicious they are.

PLANT PRODUCTS

Nuts

almonds	macadamia nuts
beech nuts	peanuts
brazil nuts	pecans
cashew nuts	pine nuts
chestnuts	pistachio nuts
coconut	walnuts
hazelnuts (filberts)	
Other	

NOTE: Leave stored nuts in their shells, and keep shelled nuts in the fridge to prevent the oils from becoming rancid. Serve them raw whenever you can and, if you do cook them, dry roast them without oil and do not add salt.

Seeds

alfalfa, lucerne (sprouted)

caraway (in cakes and bread)

coriander (as a spice)

cress (sprouted)

dill (as a spice)

fennel (as a spice, sprouted)

nutmeg

melon

mustard (as a spice and sprouted)

poppy (on bread)

pumpkin

rape (used in oil)

sesame seeds (also tahini and oil)

sunflower seeds (also oil)

Other . . . .

NOTE: You can add seeds to porridge, muesli, salads, and even to cooked vegetables. Keep them cool, as some of them contain oils that can go rancid in a warm place. To be sure of a fresh supply, do not buy them in bulk.

Sprouting seeds is the best way to grow fresh salads in your own home. Try sprouting mustard, cress, alfalfa, fennel, sesame and sunflower seeds. They are very economical; for example, a teaspoon of alfalfa seed will produce half a pound of sprouts.

Start by sowing some mustard and cress over damp tissue on the base of a plastic ice-cream box, and keep dark and just damp until the tiny shoots begin to grow (about four days); let the tiny shoots grow in the light until they make a tiny green forest, and then with a pair of scissors snip off the shoots on to a green salad. Sow every few days for a continuous supply. You will find hints, ideas and recipes for sprouted seeds, grains and beans in Leslie Kenton's book, *The Biogenic Diet* (Arrow, 1986).

Peas, beans and pulses

aduki beans

black-eyed peas

borlotti beans

broad beans

brown lentils

butter beans

chick peas

field beans

flageolet beans

French beans

garden peas

haricot beans

102

mung beans   runner beans
pinto beans   soya beans (tofu, oil)
red kidney beans   sugar peas (mangetout)
red lentils
Other ....

NOTE: These provide protein, energy, fibre and calcium in your diet, and in cold weather a good, hearty lentil and vegetable soup or bean salad will satisfy parts of you an omelette cannot reach! (See recipes, page 259 and page 272.) Dried beans and peas (pulses) make a useful winter food. The ancient Greeks sprouted them for winter salads, and so can you (see above). Pulses are the cheapest source of protein of all: their price is a little extra time to pre-soak them before cooking.

Fungi
mushrooms (various truffles
 species)
Other ....

NOTE: Unless you are an expert, never eat fungi from the wild, as they can be poisonous.

Sea vegetables
carrageen moss   seaweed
Other ....

NOTE: These are usually only available canned or dried, but look out for fresh supplies of edible seaweed in seaside areas in Wales.

Leaves
cabbage   nasturtium leaves
chicory   nettles
Chinese cabbage   parsley
chives   red cabbage
curly kale/seakale spinach
dandelion leaves   Swiss chard
globe artichoke   watercress
lettuce
Other ....

Stems

asparagus   leeks
celery
Other . . . .

Flower buds

calabrese/broccoli   cauliflower

Leaf buds

Brussels sprouts   capers
Other . . . .

Roots

beetroot	parsnip
carrots	radish
celeriac	salsify
fennel root	shallot
garlic	swede
horseradish	sweet potato
Jerusalem artichoke	turnip
kohlrabi	water chestnut
onion	yam

Other . . . .

Vegetables with seeds

cucumber   marrow
courgette, zucchini   pumpkin
gherkin   squash (various)
Other . . . .

NOTE: These vegetables have been divided up according to how they grow and which part of them we choose to eat. Try and include in your diet every day vegetables that represent all the various parts of the plant. For example, you could make a salad of lettuce (leaf), celery (stem), radish (root) and broccoli (flower). This can be another way to ensure variety and keep your diet interesting.

Wash vegetables before cooking or serving to remove traces of chemicals. Leave the skins on when you can, as many of the vitamins are found directly under the skin. Cook all vegetables in a steamer, and never cook them in advance and keep them hot, or they will lose even more of their nutrients while they are waiting.

FRUIT

Savoury fruits
avocado

olives

Tree fruits
apple (fresh, juice, cider and dried)
apricot (fresh and dried)
banana (fresh and dried)
cherry
crab apple
damson
date (fresh and dried)
fig (fresh and dried)
grapefruit (fresh, juice and dried as peel)
greengage
lemon (fresh, juice and dried as peel)
lime (juice, cordial)
lychee

mandarin orange
mango (fresh and dried)
mulberry
nectarine
orange (fresh, juice and dried as peel)
peach (fresh and dried
pear (fresh and dried)
plum (fresh or dried as prunes)
quince
satsuma/tangerine/ clementine
Seville orange
ugli fruit

Other...

Bush fruit
blackberry
blackcurrant
blueberry
cranberry
gooseberries
grapes (juice, white wine, fresh and dried as raisins, currants and sultanas)

loganberry
raspberry
redcurrant

Other...

Ground fruits

melon (e.g. galia, honeydew, watermelon)	pineapple
	rhubarb
	strawberry

Other . . . .

NOTE: Fruit is often the only raw food we eat, and as such can be the only really whole, natural food in the diet; so make sure you eat a piece of fruit at each meal, and chew it slowly and well. Wash all fruit and eat the skins on apples and pears, as they are an important source of fibre.

GRAINS AND CEREALS

barley (as pot barley, pearl barley, flakes, flour, etc.)

oats (as oatmeal, porridge, rolled oats, oatbran, etc.)

corn (as maize, sweet-corn, corn on the cob and cornflour, cornstarch, etc.)

rice (as grains, flakes, ground or flour)

rye (as flour, flakes, etc.)

Other . . . .

NOTE: These are sometimes called 'cereals', but I will call then 'grains' to distinguish them from packeted breakfast cereals. Wherever you see 'grains' referred to in the text, I am referring to this group.

Grains will be your principal source of energy on the Food Addict's Diet. They are available in a great many disguises, and all of them make good substitutes for wheat and potatoes. However, take care if you are overweight as they are high in calories.

Starch foods

arrowroot (maranta plant)

sago (sago palm root)

tapioca (cassava)

NOTE: These are unusual but easily available, and later on you will discover how useful they can be on a slimming diet (see page 181). You are more likely to find arrowroot in the chemist's shop than the supermarket – it makes a good thickener for gravies and soups.

ALTERNATIVE SUGARS AND SWEETENERS

fructose crystals   maple syrup
honey
Other . . . .

FOODS FROM MICRO-ORGANISMS

textured vegetable   yeast and yeast extract
  protein
Other . . . .

FIVE DAILY MENUS

Here are five sample menus to help you to see how the 200 foods can be used to make up a nourishing and interesting diet. I have worked out the score for each day to show you how varied your daily diet could be (see pages 70–4).

Every day you can use olive oil for salad dressing and shallow frying, and milk-free margarine to spread on oatcakes, rye crispbreads, etc. I have not included these in the variety score.

DAY 1

Breakfast
orange juice
porridge (see recipe, page 254)
fried/grilled bacon/egg/mushrooms
rye crispbread with honey
black tea or black coffee

Mid-morning snack
raw peanuts and raisins

Lunch
cold cooked chicken
crunchy salad (see recipe, page 268)
rice cakes sandwiched with honey
banana
canned mineral water with fruit juice
black tea or black coffee

Mid-afternoon snack
fresh or dried dates

Teatime snack
apple
peanuts and raisins

Supper
avocado with vinaigrette dressing (see recipe, page 267)
rabbit and bacon casserole (see recipe, page 264)
fruit salad (see recipe, page 279)

Bedtime
herbal tea or lemon and honey

(28 different ingredients eaten today)

DAY 2

Breakfast
grapefruit juice
super muesli (see recipe, page 255)
two-egg mushroom or herb omelette
rice cakes with sugar-free jam
black tea or coffee

Mid-morning snack
pear
packeted nut and seed mix

Lunch
tuna fish
tasty salad (see recipe, page 269)
rye crispbread and peanut butter
orange

Mid-afternoon snack
tropical fruit mix

Teatime snack
mineral water and apple juice
figs

Supper
chicken casserole (see recipe, page 263)
broccoli/peas/carrots
banana/grapes

Bedtime
herbal tea or lemon and honey

(36 ingredients eaten today)

DAY 3

Breakfast
pineapple juice
apple sunrise (see recipe, page 251)
kippers
rice cakes with honey
tea or coffee

Mid-morning snack
tropical fruit mix
apple

Lunch
mayonnaise salad (see recipe, page 268)
ham
oatcakes and jam

Mid-afternoon snack
sunflower seeds
raisins
mineral water

Teatime snack
tea
flapjacks (see recipe, page 283)

Supper
melon
lamb and barley hot pot (see recipe, page 264)
cabbage
carrots
green beans
apple puree with honey/raisins and flaked almonds (see recipe, page 277)

Bedtime
beef or vegetable stock drink
rye crispbreads

(35 ingredients eaten today)

DAY 4

Breakfast
pineapple juice
half grapefruit
smoked haddock with poached egg
toasted 100 per cent rye bread/sugar-free jam

Mid-morning snack
banana
cashew nuts (not salted)

Lunch
liver pâté (see recipe, page 256)

oatcakes
hard-boiled egg
crudités (see recipe, page 258)
apple

Mid-afternoon snack
figs

Teatime snack
tea or coffee
rice cakes with honey

Supper
braised pork chop (see recipe, page 263)
boiled rice
peas
sweetcorn
packeted soya dessert (see page 97)
sliced apple with raisins

Bedtime
lemon and honey drink

(28 ingredients eaten today)

DAY 5

Breakfast
pineapple juice
fried lambs' kidneys with onion and pease pudding (see
recipe, page 253)
rice cakes with tahini and honey

Mid-morning snack
banana
mineral water

Lunch
mackerel pâté (see recipe, page 256)
rye bread
carrot and celery sticks
orange and pear

Mid-afternoon snack
peanuts and raisins

Teatime snack
apple
tea with lemon and honey

Supper
celery soup (see recipe, page 260)
shepherd's parsnip pie (see recipe, page 265)
walnuts, hazelnuts, brazil nuts to crack
2 pieces of fresh fruit in season

Bedtime
vegetable stock drink
oatcakes

(26 ingredients eaten today)

This diet is very varied indeed; a total of sixty different ingredients are used during the five days. Planning in advance is vital, because the commonest reason for giving up the diet altogether, I have found, is to look in the cupboard and find that there is nothing there you are allowed to eat!

BEFORE YOU START

Now that you know what to eat we are ready to begin the four zero experiment. I suggest that you wait until next Monday, and start the diet that morning. In the meantime, let's make a note of how things stand at the moment.

I have provided space below to gather together some of the answers you gave in previous chapters, so that you will be able to compare notes conveniently at the end of the three-week experiment.

HEALTH (see page 43)

My minor symptoms at present are:

. . . .
. . . .
. . . .
. . . .

ENERGY (see page 49)

Indicate your level of energy:
Level 1: constantly tired and lacking in energy
Level 2: lack energy most of the time
Level 3: usually have enough energy for my way of life
Level 4: normally quite energetic
Level 5: abounding energy

EATING HABITS (see page 55)

(Choose one response and delete those that do not apply to you.)
I eat breakfast everyday/some days/less than twice a week/rarely/not at all.
I eat lunch every day/some days/less than twice a week/rarely/not at all.
I eat after my evening meal every day/some days/less than twice a week/rarely/not at all.
I eat snacks about . . . . times a day.
My usual snack foods are:

. . . .

YOUR PERSONAL DIET (see page 64)

Underline the phrase that best describes your personal diet:

It is: always unhealthy/sometimes unhealthy/reasonably healthy/ quite healthy/healthy/very healthy.

YOUR THREE-DAY VARIETY SCORE (see page 79)

In the three days of my food diary I ate . . . . . ingredients.

GIVING UP YOUR FAVOURITES (see page 89)

How hard would it be for you to live entirely without each of the following basic ingredients in all their various forms for just three weeks? (Draw a circle around the description that applies to you.)

Wheat	impossible/very hard/hard/easy/very easy.
Sugar	impossible/very hard/hard/easy/very easy.
Cows' milk	impossible/very hard/hard/easy/very easy.
Potatoes	impossible/very hard/hard/easy/very easy.

WHERE ARE YOU NOW?

Now you can record exactly how you feel as you set off on the diet. Do not record this information until the day before you begin.

OVERWEIGHT

Write your measurements below:
weight . . . . . st . . . . . lb (. . . . . kg)
bust/chest . . . . . in (. . . . . cm)
waist . . . . . in (. . . . . cm)
hips . . . . . in (. . . . . cm)

thighs (about 9" above knee)
   right . . . . . in (. . . . . cm)
   left . . . . . in (. . . . . cm)
upper arms
   right . . . . . in (. . . . . cm)
   left . . . . . in (. . . . . cm)

APPETITE CONTROL

This is your personal view of how good you are at controlling your intake of food. You probably call it 'will power' at the moment. There is space provided below for a personal comment to remind you of how things are.

Tick the phrase that best describes your appetite control: no control at all/very poor/poor/average/quite good/good/excellent.

Personal comment: . . . .

COPING WITH STRESS

One of the beneficial effects of the diet can be to help you deal better with stress, so make a note of how well you are coping with the stresses in your life at the moment.

Tick the phrase that best describes how well you are coping with stress: not coping at all/just managing to cope/coping reasonably well, considering/coping quite well/coping very well/absolutely no problem!

Personal comment: . . . .

SELF-CONFIDENCE

Most people who try this diet gain a great deal of self-confidence from having better appetite control.

Tick the sentence that best describes your present level of self-confidence: I have hardly any confidence in myself/I have a little confidence in myself/I am quite confident/I have no confidence problem/I am an exceptionally confident person.

Personal comment: ....

FEELINGS ABOUT YOURSELF

Make full notes here of how you feel about yourself at the moment.

....
....
....
....

You may be surprised later to see how much these feelings can change in only three weeks, so make sure to note your feelings now. Eileen, one of my diet trials participants, saw the most remarkable change in mood in just three weeks.

Eileen's first questionnaire answers told me that she suffered cravings for food, a lack of will power, chronic tiredness and a lack of self-confidence. Her personal remarks before she began the diet were:

'I feel disgust – I don't want to go out. I have let my appearance go because whatever I wear I know it doesn't look good, so I am inclined not to bother at all. I feel like hiding away, and dread being in company. I don't even want to go to work.'

Just four weeks later Eileen was 7 pounds lighter, and her second questionnaire told a very different story:

'There has been a great change in my general well-being. I have shaken off tiredness, no energy, lethargy, general feelings of debility and aching joints and bones. I feel much more able to cope. Before going on the diet, I was struggling to cope with my work by lunchtime, but now it is not a problem. I was very irritable and snappy and on the verge of leaving home before I started eating your way, but all that has passed now.'

When I read that questionnaire, I knew that I had found a diet that could change lives: I hope it will do the same for you when you try the three-week four zero experiment.

CHAPTER 7
The Four Zero Experiment

The whole experiment takes just over four weeks and consists of three stages: exactly three weeks following the zero plan, four days on the rest test, and five days on the restart plan. You will find details of the rest test and the restart plan in Chapter 8. This chapter deals exclusively with the details of the first three weeks on the zero plan.

THE ZERO PLAN

You will follow a diet that:

1. Avoids all traces of cows' milk, beet and cane sugar, wheat and potatoes (see pages 17–37).

2. Only includes alcohol in the form of dry white wine and cider (see page 60).

3. Avoids salt as far as possible (see page 61).

4. Avoids refined or hydrogenated oils as far as possible (see page 63).

5. Includes at least a litre of fluid a day (see page 58).

6. Consists wherever possible of real, whole food in as much variety as you can afford, chosen from the list of 200 foods on pages 98–107.

FOLLOWING THE PLAN

The experiment falls into four stages:

1. The first four days when you are getting used to it.

2. The end of the first week when you discover the magic of this way of eating.

3. The second week when you find that social pressures begin to get in the way of your new diet.

4. The third week when you will either be feeling complacent or very deprived, depending on how much of an addict you are!

'I can't do it!'

At any time during this process you may break the rules, just for a taste of one of the four zeros. This could make you feel a failure and you may then want to give up altogether. You are addicted to food and not lacking will power, so keep trying! Relax, read the whole of this chapter and the next, and see how the restart plan (page 136) can help you to make a new beginning.

STAGE 1: THE FIRST FOUR DAYS

You will find that practically no effort is required to begin the experiment, because you can eat as much as you like at meal times and in between.

Tips for success

Use the recipes on pages 245–85 or the daily menus on pages 107–12 for ideas about what to eat. The meals can be mixed according to your personal needs, or you can use the menus as a set diet plan if that is what you prefer.

Do not ration yourself: you will feel very hungry and deprived during the first few days. In fact, your addictive cravings may overwhelm your will power many times, and there will probably be many false starts before you get going properly.

Take it easy, and if you are hungry, then eat! As far as possible, let your body decide when it wants to eat, not your clock. However, even if you normally don't eat breakfast, try to eat something before 10 o'clock in the morning every day. The food you are now eating will not

initially seem so satisfying and you will feel deprived.
You can cope with this by having frequent snacks of
allowed food. Remember, this is not 'true' hunger but an
addictive craving (see pages 91–2).

Withdrawal symptoms

If you started to feel below par the day after you began
the plan, and have developed all kinds of mysterious
symptoms, then you have made your first step: withdrawal symptoms are positive proof that your previous
diet has been affecting your health.

Common symptoms of withdrawal are: headaches and
migraines; extreme tiredness; lethargy; aching limbs;
dizziness; digestive upset: flatulence, stomach ache,
diarrhoea; sore or dry throat; cold or runny nose; disturbed sleep.

Withdrawal symptoms can be eased by drinking plenty
of fluids and eating plenty of raw vegetables and fruits.
Do not exert yourself too much, get plenty of rest, take
gentle exercise out of doors, and wait for the symptoms
to pass.

Marie's first four days on the plan

Marie was a trials participant in 1988, and this chapter
will follow her experiences during the experiment. A
mother of three, she lives on a farm and was about one
stone overweight at the start of the experiment. Here is
an extract from a report she wrote for me about her first
four days on the plan:

'At first the mere thought of giving up the four zeros
was startling – giving up either bread or potatoes would
have been OK, but not both! Being a nibbler I found it
hard at first to make the children sandwiches without
picking at a piece of bread or cheese.

'I do not usually eat breakfast, because it seems to
stimulate my appetite and then I want to eat all day, but
I have managed a little fruit about 9.30 or 10.00 every
morning this week. I don't enjoy black tea and can't get
on with the taste of soya milk, so I stick to black coffee.

By about 8 p.m. my tummy feels really bloated and uncomfortable, and probably due to the high fibre content of this diet I have a wind problem!' (This is due to withdrawal.)

STAGE 2: THE END OF THE FIRST WEEK

On the fifth day of the experiment there will not be a single trace of the zero foods in your body, because they will have worked their way through your intestines and cannot bother you any more. Now you can begin to discover the magic of the Food Addict's Diet.

Marie's magic Friday
Here is Marie's report written on her first Friday on the plan:

'Although my calorie intake must be lower, I have not felt at all hungry. I have not been bored or wanted to cheat. Usually diets begin on Monday and finish on Wednesday at the latest! I get frequent headaches, but I haven't had one all week. I've got more energy: I used to feel tired by 7 p.m. but now I can keep going rather than flopping into a chair in front of the TV.

'Not eating the zero foods was easier than I had anticipated. Monday and Tuesday were easy: on Wednesday I had to keep really busy to avoid temptation, Thursday was encouraging because I felt so well and energetic, but today, Friday, was marvellous!'

Experiences on the experiment do vary from person to person, but I noticed a set of five particular improvements that I have called the 'magic' of this change of diet.

Five kinds of magic

1. Reduced hunger, increased will power
After three days or so on the plan your hunger diminishes, because those addictive cravings have gone: they have been starved of the very foods that kept them alive, and have simply died. Now your natural hunger can take over

120

control of your eating. It was once overwhelmed by your cravings, but now it is controlled without using any will power at all. Now you can resist foods that would have once been your downfall and it is all much easier than you ever thought possible.

2. A good feeling

One day this week you will wake up feeling really well, perhaps better than for years. On this day, usually about the fifth day of the experiment, you will feel an unexpected sense of lightness and clarity, as though seeing the world for the first time. It feels so good that it will make the struggle of the first few days well worth while.

This feeling of almost lightheaded euphoria can persist for more than a week and there might be a slight 'let-down' in the third week (see pages 125–6). Even so, the light and clear feeling remains and will keep you feeling good for as long as you continue to avoid the zero foods.

3. Extra energy

By the end of the first week you will notice that you have more energy. This is not the kind that sends you into a turmoil of frantic activity, turning out filing cabinets and spring-cleaning wardrobes: it is a slow, more dependable supply that is always there when you need it. You won't have to drag yourself to work or force yourself to do things – you will just find yourself doing them! For weary housewives plodding through the days, this is magic indeed!

4. Symptoms improved

There can be an improvement in symptoms even in the first week: less pain in the joints, fewer headaches, less indigestion, etc. For those constantly troubled by debilitating minor symptoms, this may be the first real relief for many years.

5. A feeling of quiet confidence

Notice how much better you are sleeping, how much more patient you are with your family, and how much better you are at coping with the stresses in your life. One-time guilty eaters now free of guilt and self-blame can begin to feel more confident. This sudden increase in confidence feels very fragile and unreliable at first, but gradually you can begin to take it for granted and start making new decisions and changes. This is how this diet changes lives, and it is the greatest magic of all.

The first weekend

If you live a very different life on weekdays, your first weekend on the plan will present a new challenge. The family is around you, friends drop in, you are invited out, there may be a party or a wedding, and there are the traditions of the Sunday lunch to cope with. That pressure to conform will be at its strongest, so be ready.

Remind yourself of what you have gained already, and tell yourself not to risk losing all that control just for the sake of eating the same way as everybody else. Use your new-found confidence to hold out against this pressure to conform.

Plan exactly what to eat that first weekend, and make sure that there is plenty for the family or visitors too. If you are entertaining at home, make foods that you can enjoy. If you eat out, make sure you are not too hungry by having a small snack before you go.

Stick to white wine only: no red wine, remember. This may be the first alcohol you have taken this week, so be wary if you have an eating problem, as alcohol triggers an eating binge faster than any food! (See the hints on pages 206–8 for dealing with a binge.)

If you invite some friends around to eat, use some recipes from this book and provide the zero foods separately, just for them. If you want to hide the fact that you are on a diet, this way your friends will never guess!

If you just cannot stick to the rules at a dinner party, don't despair. If you find pastry or potato on your plate and you can't avoid it, at least enjoy it! However, don't be surprised to find your cravings awakened by the next morning!

STAGE 3: THE SECOND WEEK – FINDING NEW PLEASURES

The second week will feel quite different from the first. You are now an expert on what to eat, and this new diet is almost second nature already. The plan is no longer a problem to follow, and the idea of crispbreads and soya milk no longer feels so outlandish.

As time passes there is an increasing possibility that something will happen to make you break the rules and take some of the zero foods. The effects of doing this can be quite dramatic, sometimes taking the form of a full-scale return of your usual symptoms, or even some new ones. If you break down badly, turn to the restart plan on pages 136–8 to get you going again.

For some people the second week is a kind of plateau where nothing seems to be happening, and the temptation is to give up. If you feel this way, keep going, for when you come to your second assessment on page 126 you may be surprised at the results!

For most people, like Marie, there is a steady improvement throughout the week, maintained by the prevailing positive mood.

Marie's second week

By the second week Marie was eating a little more for breakfast. Her initial wind problem passed at about the time when her bowel movements became more consistent: she had oscillated from constipation to very loose motions for the first few days.

This is her report:

'The next week was easy. I found that I was into a routine now and managed OK except for the office party on Friday, which I was dreading. I managed to refuse a Danish pastry on Wednesday and a pizza on Thursday. On Thursday I told them at the office that I was on a diet to test for food intolerance, and they were so interested! For the party I brought in some special flapjacks and oat-cakes and pâté as my contribution, and they loved them.

'During the second weekend we stayed with some friends in Derby and I had to eat normally, but I did not have as much as usual and genuinely didn't want seconds! It felt good not to be bloated after Sunday lunch.

'I was a lot hungrier on the Monday after all that food, and I had my first headache since starting the plan, but it passed by the afternoon. Oddly enough, I don't feel guilty about giving in like I used to. I have lost eight pounds, and I can't believe I am nearly there!'

Learning to cope

Marie knew that she could not resist the cakes and crisps at the office party, and she did not want to let the party spoil her diet, so she did two very sensible things. First, she told her associates that she was on a special diet for food intolerance, and secondly, she took in a contribution that would satisfy her hunger and show her friends that the plan is not a faddy and peculiar diet. Follow Marie's example and you will be able to stick to the plan and not be labelled a 'health freak'!

Finding new rewards

Marie has found new rewards to replace the pleasure once obtained from her food: the feeling of control that she felt when she was able to refuse the pastry and the pizza was every bit as good as the pleasure she once gained from eating it!

Once a 'good blow-out' was a pleasure, but now Marie prefers to feel satisfied than to be full-up, weighed down by the food in her stomach and only capable of a nap after lunch! Her true hunger has taken control at last, and she finds it much easier to keep her food consumption at a reasonable, healthy level.

Marie's experience on the Monday illustrates how her attitude has changed to breaking her diet intentions. Once she would have given up in despair having broken her diet, but this time she was surprised to find that for once there was no guilt and no despair.

STAGE 4: THE THIRD WEEK – ENTHUSIASM BEGINS TO WANE

If you are lucky, you will sail through this week unscathed, but for most people the real problems begin now. You have been on the diet long enough to have forgotten what it felt like before, and that initial euphoric feeling is beginning to fade.

All around you other people seem to be enjoying themselves, happily eating foods now denied to you. The social pressure to conform is at its strongest now, as the 'old days' of two weeks ago when nothing was restricted or forbidden become bathed in a rosy glow. This is an important low point, and if you are to cope with it successfully, you must see it for what it is: – just another step in overcoming your addiction to food.

Feeling deprived

This is stage 5 of overcoming your addiction to food (see page 88), so recognise the feeling for what it is. You are of course not deprived of food because you are getting three good meals a day: you are missing the lift the four zero foods used to bring you. You used them to carry you through each day's minor crises, but you no longer have that prop. Realise that it is not food you need, but some relief from stress and strain, so try to make each day interesting but not exhausting, and get enough proper rest.

Jeannie: Deprived of milk

Jeannie, a West Indian mother of five and clearly a milk addict from her reports, phoned me one night in her third week and complained about a 'constant hungry feeling in her stomach' that was keeping her awake at night. She said she was missing the hot milk she used to drink before bed, and was unable to sleep well without it. She said it had not been a problem in the first week, but had gradually increased since the middle of the second, so it was clearly not a craving, but a feeling of being

125

deprived of comfort. I suggested various drinks as a substitute, and the very best was camomile tea, sweetened
with honey. Once she discovered how soothing and
relaxing this was, she slept well and was able to continue
happily with the plan.

Two ways to keep things interesting

Keep your diet varied
It is very important to maintain interest in your food
during this week, and to keep your daily diet varied. If
you are bored with the diet then you are not trying hard
enough to make it interesting. Don't slap milk-free margarine on Ryvita and call it lunch: make it a good meal.
Keep your score as high as you can and make full use of
the recipe section in this book on pages 245–85.

Make a second food diary
Record your food over three consecutive days in the
third week as you did before starting the plan (p. 79),
calculate your variety score again, and see how much it
has risen in just three weeks.

My three days total variety score is . . . . . ingredients

HOW WAS IT FOR YOU?

Congratulations! You have reached the end of your
three weeks on the zero plan. The next step is to see how
the diet has affected your health and appetite.

Now you can fill in the following form and then compare it with the form on pages 113–16 to see how much
things have changed in the three weeks.

HEALTH

My minor symptoms now are:
a . . . .
b . . . .

c ....
d ....
e ....

How much have they improved? Put a circle around the words/word that best describes your symptoms now:

a) Worse/the same/a little better/very much better/ completely disappeared.
b) Worse/the same/a little better/very much better/ completely disappeared.
c) Worse/the same/a little better/very much better/ completely disappeared.
d) Worse/the same/a little better/very much better/ completely disappeared.

ENERGY

Indicate your present level of energy:
Level 1: constantly tired and lacking in energy
Level 2: lack energy most of the time
Level 3: usually have enough energy for my way of life
Level 4: normally quite energetic
Level 5: abounding energy

EATING HABITS

I eat breakfast every day/some days/less than twice a week/rarely/not at all.
I eat lunch every day/some days/less than twice a week/ rarely/not at all.
I eat after my evening meal every day/some days/less than twice a week/rarely/not at all.
I eat snacks about .... times a day.
My usual snack foods are:

....

YOUR PERSONAL DIET

Underline the phrase that best describes your personal diet now: Always unhealthy/sometimes unhealthy/reasonably healthy/quite healthy/healthy/very healthy.

YOUR SECOND THREE-DAY VARIETY SCORE (see page 114)

In the three days of my second food diary I ate .....
ingredients.

GIVING UP YOUR FAVOURITES

How hard was it living entirely without the four zeros for three weeks?
(Circle the description that applies to you.)

Wheat was	impossible/very hard/hard/easy/very easy
Sugar was	impossible/very hard/hard/easy/very easy
Cows' milk was	impossible/very hard/hard/easy/very easy
Potatoes were	impossible/very hard/hard/easy/very easy

OVERWEIGHT

Write your present measurements below:
date: ....
weight ..... st ..... lb (..... kg)
bust/chest ..... in (..... cm)
waist ..... in (..... cm)
hips ..... in (..... cm)
thighs (about 9" above knee)
   right ..... in (..... cm)
   left ..... in (..... cm)
upper arms

right ..... in (..... cm)
left ..... in (..... cm)

APPETITE CONTROL

Circle the phrase that best describes your appetite control at present: No control at all/very poor/poor/average/quite good/good/excellent.
Personal comment: ....

COPING WITH STRESS

Circle the phrase that best describes how well you are coping with stress at the moment: not coping at all/just managing to cope/coping reasonably well, considering/coping quite well/coping very well/absolutely no problem!

Personal comment: ....

SELF-CONFIDENCE

Circle the sentence that best describes your present level of self-confidence: I have hardly any confidence in myself/I have a little confidence in myself/I am quite confident/I have no confidence problem/I am an exceptionally confident person.

Personal comment: ....

FEELINGS ABOUT YOURSELF

Make full notes here of how you feel about yourself at the moment.
....
....
....
....
....

THE RESULTS

I can only hope the results of the experiment were as good for you as they were for the 100 people who applied to try the diet in 1988–9.

Here are some of the results:

SYMPTOMS

The symptoms that were most improved were headaches, depression, lethargy, arthritic pain, irritability, indigestion and fluid retention. Obviously this was coupled with a decrease in the need for drugs, mainly pain killers and antacid tablets.

ENERGY

The commonest reported improvement during the trials was an increase in energy, from which all kinds of other improvements were derived: more outdoor exercise, more sport, and a more active existence generally – which is good news for anyone who wants to lose weight.

EATING HABITS

Candidates tended to increase their consumption of water (52 per cent), fruit (63 per cent), vegetables (53 per cent), fish (43 per cent) and meat (37 per cent). Some 36 per cent of the candidates drank less alcohol and 54 per cent drank less tea and coffee.

There was a marked move towards eating breakfast – and cooked breakfast in particular (35 per cent). There was little change to lunchtime eating habits, but 54 per cent ate less often after the evening meal during the plan.

THE VARIETY SCORE

Among the fifty candidates who completed the diaries, the first scores were very low, averaging only 19.3. The second diary, with four major food ingredients missing, showed a definite increase to an average of 22.6. There was one woman who had a score of only 8 for one day before the plan, which increased to 16 in one day three weeks later – a 100 per cent improvement in variety.

GIVING UP THE FOUR ZEROS

When asked how difficult it was to give up the four foods, the following responded with 'very difficult', 'difficult' or 'hard' on their questionnaires: milk 54 per cent, wheat 42 per cent, potatoes 31 per cent, and sugar 22 per cent. Very few (11 per cent) managed to predict correctly the foods they would find hardest to give up. Many said afterwards that they were surprised how easy it all was, despite their fears at the beginning!

We have now come to the end of your three weeks on the four zero plan and you should have a much clearer idea of your relationship to your food. We have another two steps to take before the four zero experiment is over: the rest test and the restart plan. The restart plan sets this diet apart from all the others, because it will teach you how to succeed by learning to cope with your failures. To find out what you must do, turn to Chapter 8.

CHAPTER 8
Rest and Restart

Now you have come to the end of your three weeks on the four zero plan, you are almost ready for Part Three, when you will be able to apply what you have learned to build yourself a special diet to solve your particular problem – whether excess weight, food intolerance symptoms or poor appetite control. However, no diet book can possibly be complete without instructions to be followed in the event of diet breakdown, and this chapter will provide them.

Any diet plan can come to an end prematurely when a moment of weakness leads to total diet breakdown and the accompanying feeling of failure and hopelessness that makes things much worse. You may have already experienced this problem several times on various diets, even this one.

Your three weeks on the plan will have already provided an answer to diet breakdown, because you will have noticed in the first week how quickly you can have your cravings under control with the help of the four zero plan. If you do lapse from the plan and allow your old bad eating habits to reassert themselves, that wonderful feeling of control can soon be yours again if you simply begin again and wait just four days for your cravings to die.

However, the first time you taste those four zero foods after your first three weeks without them you may misunderstand the surge of hunger you feel and your sudden lack of control. If you despair then of ever being able to begin again, your three weeks on the plan will all be wasted. This is what happened to Tricia, one of the first guinea pigs to try the four zero plan, and I introduced the rest test and the restart plan as part of the experiment to help her to cope with that feeling of despair and make a new start.

Tricia

Tricia carefully followed her three weeks on the plan without deviating from it once, and continued with it for another three weeks because she found it an excellent way to lose weight. After six weeks she had lost 14 pounds and had reached her correct weight. Then she began to wonder how she was to eat in the future to maintain her new slim figure.

I told her that she could adapt the plan to keep her slim for life, but that she might like gradually to introduce the banned foods into her diet again. Because of her enthusiasm, she had not eaten a scrap of the four banned foods for six weeks, but as soon as she started to eat them again she could not stop!

After all those weeks of very successful slimming and having almost reached her target weight, she returned to her old ways. She became withdrawn and depressed, and her weight shot up rapidly by over a stone until it was higher than it had been before. Try as I might, I could not persuade her to begin again for a long time.

Tricia had thought that somehow the mere fact of being slim would keep her food consumption down for ever, and she felt really bad about giving in after so many weeks of being in control. Her despair was rooted in the idea that she was basically greedy, for once she tasted the four zeros again her hunger increased markedly as her cravings were reawakened, and this is what she thought was her greedy nature reasserting itself.

Clearly, Tricia needed a further exercise to help her to understand that sudden surge of hunger. First of all, we followed another three weeks on the plan as before and

Tricia was glad to feel her cravings die down in the first four days. This time I insisted that after the first three weeks she should deliberately take a rest from the plan and keep a diary of what she ate while noticing how her cravings increased. After a few days' rest she began the plan again and observed her cravings dying away.

This is how Tricia discovered the secret of the Food Addict's Diet: that anyone can switch their cravings on and off according to what they eat, and that it has nothing to do with will power or greed. Tricia remained on the plan for a further eight weeks, and lost weight again, just as easily as before. She now carefully avoids sugar and milk, both of which she finds very tempting, and in this way she keeps her eating under control to maintain her new slim figure.

TRYING TO BE PERFECT

On the trials there were a few candidates who decided that they were hopeless cases because they could not stick to the plan for every day of the whole three weeks and 'be perfect', and the slightest mistake sent them into despair.

The Food Addict's Diet recognises that nobody's perfect: this diet is simply about learning to cope with your cravings through good times and bad, and the rest test and restart plan are an important part of that learning process.

With a little help from Rudyard Kipling I put together these few words of counsel for the bad times: *'If I can keep my head when all about me are the foods I love; if I can see that a slight mistake is not the end of the world; if I can pick myself up and start again as often as it takes – then one day I will win.'*

REST AND RESTART

The four-day rest test and the five-day restart plan make up a kind of rehearsal for those times when your diet will break down and you will need to make a new start.

During the nine days of rest and restart you will be able to observe all of the physical effects of diet breakdown but without the feelings of failure, guilt or despair. Once you have learned how to keep your head and simply start again instead of blaming yourself you will have a useful strategy to help you get back on top whenever your dieting intentions begin to fade.

THE REST TEST

This is quite simply four days off the diet. Eat whatever you fancy and forget about slimming and food intolerance for a while, but take careful note of what you choose to eat and drink. Make a food diary as before (see page 75) and include *every* occasion during the day when you ate a zero food in any form. You do not need to record the other foods this time.

How many times altogether did you take the following foods each day?

Day 1
wheat   . . . times
milk   . . . times
sugar   . . . times
potatoes   . . . times

Day 2
wheat   . . . times
milk   . . . times
sugar   . . . times
potatoes   . . . times

Day 3
wheat   . . . times
milk   . . . times
sugar   . . . times
potatoes   . . . times

Day 4

wheat   ... times
milk   ... times
sugar   ... times
potatoes ... times

On this day also make a careful note of your symptoms, your mood and your weight. Notice how much your mood and weight have altered, and now you know exactly why!

WHICH ZERO IS YOUR FIX?

Notice which of the zeros you ate most often during the four-day rest test. This is the food you find most tempting, and is probably also the one that you eat first when you break your diet. This food always gives you a pleasant sense of satisfaction, and when you are feeling a bit low, it helps to cheer you up – it is, in fact, your fix! Notice which foods you cannot control, and remember what you have learned, for this is the key to permanent weight control!

THE RESTART PLAN

This is nothing more than a repeat of the first four days of the experiment. When you wake up on the fifth day you will be back to that positive state of mind you possessed in the first week, and with your new sense of confidence and control you will be ready to stay with the diet for as long as it takes to solve your particular problem.

A DAY AT A TIME

Before you start again
Make sure than you have plenty of the allowed foods in the house. Plan ahead what you are going to eat in the

next few days. Use the recipes on pages 245–85 and shop for substitutes.

The first day
Be gentle on yourself. Do not tell yourself that you must eat less as a sort of 'punishment' for eating the banned foods during the rest test. You are beginning again, right from the start, and what happened yesterday is not important – think of today. Expect to feel very hungry today, so enjoy three good meals and snacks whenever you need them.

The second day
Three more days seems a long time to wait for the 'magic' of the diet to return, and you may already be giving up hope. Keep going, for all those negative feelings will pass if you persevere. If you gained weight during the three-day rest test, you may be tempted to limit your food intake, but don't do that. Just keep eating good, satisfying meals, for you have the rest of your life to undo any damage.

The zero foods will seem tempting still, so let yourself have plenty of allowed nibbles. Eat a good, high-protein, high-vegetable diet today. Drink plenty of water and take extra Vitamin C if you get withdrawal symptoms. If you have a withdrawal headache, Vitamin C will help more than aspirin.

The third day
The last of the zero foods you ate three days ago will leave your body at some time today, and you will begin to feel better.

The fourth day
You should be feeling brighter and better, and if you just keep calm and avoid the four zeros, you will make it.

Fifth day: Back on top!

On the morning of the fifth day, you should be feeling in charge of yourself again. Your weight should have dropped a little, and you should feel ready for anything.

Samantha: A happy ending

Samantha, an unmarried mother with a young baby, was one of the last to try the three weeks on the four zero plan. During the experiment, she found herself better able to cope with the strains of bringing up a baby on her own, but she did not see how it could be related to her diet.

However, after the four-day rest test she was amazed at the change in her mood: a minor argument with her boyfriend on the second rest day developed into a crashing row which went on into the night. She felt very low and irritable, and her skin became greasier. She discovered that she took milk twenty times over the four days' rest, mainly in the form of cheese and yoghurt. She had always thought she must be a cheese addict, and this confirmed it.

She began the restart plan, and within three days she was much calmer and brighter and was able to see that her boyfriend was being quite reasonable after all. At last she could see clearly the effect of food on her mood as well as on her weight. They married four months later, and Samantha lost her excess weight (10 pounds) in time for the wedding.

WHAT NEXT?

The rest test has pinpointed for you the food you find hardest to control, and there may be more than one. These are best avoided, but if there are any that you do not seem to be addicted to and you can control your intake, why not try eating them?

Joan brings back milk and sugar

Joan (whose story you read on page 85) found it remarkably easy to avoid milk products and to refuse sweets and chocolate while on the zero plan. However, she could not

138

resist potatoes and wheat, and every time her diet broke down it was bread or biscuits that tempted her and reawakened her cravings.

During her rest test she took milk products seven times, sugary food four times, potato products four times but wheat-based food fifteen times! This confirmed what she already knew – that she was a wheat addict. Although she only ate potatoes once or twice a day, she always wanted to eat them in their skins and ate the skins too. She loves potato crisps made with whole jacket potatoes and has decided that she must be a little bit addicted to the solanine which is concentrated in the skin of potatoes (see page 35).

She decided that milk and sugar could safely return, in small doses, for she found that she was able to exercise restraint in dealing with foods such as ice cream or yoghurt. This left potatoes and wheat, so she decided to avoid potato skins but eat the rest of the potato and avoid all wheat for ever. This formula suits her perfectly and is now her everyday diet.

BRINGING BACK SOME OF THE FOUR ZEROS

If you want to do the same as Joan, introduce each zero food singly for a few days, and take good note of its effects on your weight and appetite, etc. Then return to the plan for at least a week and try another zero food, until you have tried them all. By then you will know which of the zeros, you must avoid for ever and which can be taken in small doses.

You may find that your symptoms return when you take some of the four zero foods again; for advice about what to do about this, see chapter 11. Perhaps all four of the zero foods awaken your cravings whenever you take them; in that case you have multiple addictions, and you will need to stay on the plan for a very long time and make frequent use of the restart plan to keep your cravings under control.

BRINGING BACK ALL OF THE FOUR ZEROS

If you found that you could give up the four zeros easily, that you were not suddenly attracted to them on the rest test and you had no particular health problems to overcome, then at least the experiment will have shown you how repetitive the British diet can be. However, you will know how to eat foods in greater variety than before, which can only be beneficial to your health.

USING THE PLAN FOR SPECIAL PROBLEMS

The zero plan forms the basis of three types of diet: a slimming diet, an elimination diet and a healthy eating diet. Part Three will help you to adapt the four zero plan to suit your needs exactly, whatever your problem, but before you turn to the next chapter make sure that you are free of all cravings for the four zeros by completing at least five days of the four zero plan. Then you will be ready to use the Food Addict's Diet to deal with your particular problem, which is most likely to be the greatest health problem of our modern age: being overweight.

Part Three
After the Experiment

CHAPTER 9
Losing Weight for Good with the Food Addict's Diet

Now that you have tried the four zero experiment you will have discovered that your excess weight is the result of your unnatural appetite for high-calorie foods. This chapter is based on this and two other important facts about being overweight. First, you can slim and stay healthy on any slimming diet if you eat healthy food and stick to the diet for long enough. Secondly, it is possible for anyone to eat a good, filling, nourishing diet every day without gaining weight. In this chapter we will develop all these ideas into a strategy to help you to slim and stay slim.

Many of you will have lost a considerable amount of weight already by simply adopting the four zero plan as your daily diet, and you are probably quite content to remain on the plan until your weight reaches the correct level. You have lost weight because you automatically reduced your food intake when your hunger diminished.

If you continued to eat a lot of substitute high-calorie foods on the plan, you probably lost a little weight at first and then stabilised: you will need to reduce your food intake further to begin losing weight. If you lost no weight at all on the experiment, do not despair! You will be able to with the help of the ideas in this chapter.

THE PLAN AS A MAINTENANCE DIET

Every time you lose weight on a slimming diet you are probably haunted by the fear of ending up back where you started once you resume normal eating. To prevent weight gain you need a healthy, satisfying maintenance diet comprised of easily available foods. You now know what this is – it is the Food Addict's Diet!

A remarkable effect of the experiment worth mentioning here is that among the 100 people on the diet trials nobody gained weight, although I set no artificial limits or restrictions on the amount of food consumed. This way of eating may not act as a weight-loss regime for everyone, but it certainly makes an excellent weight-maintenance plan.

SIX SLIMMING OPTIONS

We are all very different and respond to weight-loss programmes in various ways, so in the following pages I suggest six different slimming options, all based on the plan.

All six slimming options assume that you remain on the plan throughout, for eliminating all the zero foods from your diet must be at the heart of your slimming effort – even those foods you find easy to control. Remember that this also includes taking alcohol only in the form of white wine and cider. While you are slimming you should take no more than two glasses a day, and preferably none at all.

The first two options are based on an important maxim: food addicts manage a diet better if they completely avoid a food than if they set out to reduce consumption of it.

OPTION 1: NO GRAINS

Most of the heavily overweight candidates on the trials had a strong appetite for all grain-based foods. They found wheat the hardest of the four zero foods to avoid during the experiment and unearthed all manner of substitute breads and cookies to enjoy. Most of them normally experienced digestive disorders such as bloating and constipation, and many of them developed either flatulence or slight diarrhoea as a withdrawal symptom in the first few days of the plan. These symptoms are also signs of food intolerance (see pages 41–3) so it seems that many overweight people are intolerant of grain-based foods.

These grain-sensitive candidates seemed to retain fluid, which they lost rapidly in the first week of the plan. Their stomachs tended to be distended, which became worse in the first week of the plan with the introduction of other cereals. The candidates who suffered in this way found the grain-free option most effective.

With the grain-free option the following foods are banned:

The four zeros:
Wheat; cows' milk; beet and cane sugar; potatoes.

The seven grains:
Rye; barley; oats; rice; corn; wheat; millet.

The following foods are *allowed* on the grain-free option:

meats	arrowroot
fish	tapioca
eggs	sago
beans	honey and other
peas	sweeteners
nuts	olive oil
seeds	white wine and cider
dried and fresh fruit	(not more than two
vegetables	glasses per day)

Avoid fatty meats where you can, but make sure you eat olive oil, nuts and seeds to obtain the fatty acids, for they are important in metabolising body fat.

145

Making a start

If you have not been following the plan when you begin this option, then start first by cutting out the four zeros on the restart plan (see pages 136–8), and on the fifth day start eliminating the seven grains. If you are a grain addict, you may feel extremely hungry and deprived at first and suffer withdrawal symptoms, such as diarrhoea or headache, but this will pass in another two or three days.

Your body and your appetite will have calmed down completely about five days after you give up the other grains, and you will find you want to eat much less than usual. With a smaller appetite to match your smaller food consumption, you should find this option easy to follow and your weight decreasing gradually at an average rate of about two pounds a week.

Gracie goes grain-free

Gracie was one of my favourite guinea pigs! She was seventy-five years old when she tried the experiment. She could not walk far owing to an arthritic hip, and was three stones overweight. Her doctor had told her three months previously to lose those three stones in time for another operation.

When she approached me to try the diet, Gracie had managed to cut her food down enough to lose a stone, but she had another two stones to lose. She followed the experiment, but only lost two pounds. She then tried going grain-free, and after two weeks she told me: 'I still take no exercise, I feel as if I am eating three times my normal amount but I have still lost seven pounds!'

This was the most generous slimming diet that Gracie had ever tried. She was losing weight while eating three good meals a day. Her last three-stone major slimming effort had required hospitalisation on 600 calories a day. By following my no-grains regime for twelve weeks, Gracie lost nearly two stones while eating well, and her second operation has now taken place.

Some people become quite neurotic when they try

deliberately to limit their food intake, and suffer relapses in their appetite control that take weeks to repair. If you are like this, try the no-grains option to lose weight without tears, because you can eat as much as you like as long as you avoid the zero foods and all the grains. This option does not feel like a normal slimming diet, as one can tuck into naughty sweet snacks such as dates, figs, seeds or raisins without guilt. This is by far the easiest option to follow if you enjoy your food!

OPTION 2: THE 'SLIM WEEK'

Everyone on the diet trials found that they eventually reached a certain weight from which it was difficult to move. The 'slim week' is a planned, concerted effort to cut food down for one week only, after which almost anyone can expect a weight loss of at least three pounds. At the end of the week you return to the basic plan as a maintenance diet.

If you are a grain addict, try this three-week diet cycle for an effective way to lose weight without getting bored or suffering too much:

Week one: No grains
Week two: No grains
Week three: Slim week

Then revert to the basic plan for a while to maintain your weight loss until you feel ready to try a further slimming effort.

Before you start, here are some tips to help you succeed in the 'slim week' plan:

1. Notice that there are NO grains, animal milks, sugars or dried fruits allowed.
2. Take meals at these times:
   Breakfast: before 10.30 a.m.
   Lunch: between 11.45 a.m. and 3 p.m.
   Evening meal: between 5.00 p.m. and 8.00 p.m.
3. Try to have as many different foods as possible in

the week, and vary the vegetables from day to day.

4. Don't leave the oil out of your diet this week. Use small amounts of olive oil to fry or grill meat, to make vinaigrette for salads or make home-made mayonnaise. Serve all salads with one tablespoon of fresh mayonnaise or two tablespoons of vinaigrette or French dressing (see recipes, pages 266–7).

5. As so many calcium-rich foods are removed, it is essential that you take a calcium supplement this week.

6. The days and meals can be interchanged to fit in with your week. Try to keep to one salad meal and one cooked meal a day, or you will soon get bored!

7. If you have to eat out during the week, simply eat what is given but avoid the zero foods wherever possible. Do not use a meal out as an excuse to give up the 'slim week'.

8. If you have to change the menus because you don't like the foods I have suggested, remember not to eat any grains or other starch foods, dried fruits or animal milk products while on the 'slim week'.

9. If you are vegetarian, instead of meats or fish choose a whole-protein combination of seeds or nuts with beans or pulses (and eggs if you eat them). Vary the combinations and ingredients as much as possible – e.g. walnuts and lima beans, peanuts and sunflower seeds.

10. The following hot drinks are allowed in any quantity and at any time of day while on the 'slim week': herb teas; black tea; black coffee; vegetable stock drink (stir one teaspoonful of vegetable-stock paste into a mug of hot water).

THE 'SLIM WEEK' MENUS

DAY ONE

On rising
2 glasses of mineral water

Breakfast
fruit salad
(chop 2 fresh fruits into a little fruit juice)
4 oz/100 g kippers poached in water
1 glass of fruit juice
black tea or coffee

Mid-morning
1 glass of fruit juice
black tea or coffee
1 whole fruit

Lunch
4 oz/100 g cold lean meat
tasty salad (see recipe, page 269)
1 glass fruit juice
black tea or coffee

Mid-afternoon
2 glasses of mineral water
1 whole fruit

Evening meal
omelette made with 2 eggs and mixed herbs and 2 tsps of
 olive oil
selection of green vegetables lightly cooked

Bedtime
any amount of allowed hot drink

DAY 2

(Easy-pack lunch, slow-cook evening meal)

On rising
2 glasses of mineral water

Breakfast
1 whole grapefruit, peeled and chopped
2 rashers of lean back bacon fried lightly in 2 tsps olive

oil with 3 mushrooms sliced and fried in same pan
1 glass of fruit juice

Mid-morning
2 glasses fruit juice

Lunch
4 oz/100 g canned tuna or salmon (in brine)
large crunchy salad (see recipes, page 268)
1 glass fruit juice

Mid-afternoon
2 glasses mineral water
1 whole fruit

Evening meal
1 large or 2 small lamb chops braised in olive oil with
    onion
celery and carrot with herbs and seasonings
green vegetables lightly cooked
mineral water to drink with meal

Bedtime
any amount of allowed hot drink

DAY 3

(Quick-cook lunch, easy-to-serve evening meal)

On rising
2 glasses of mineral water

Breakfast
1 large slice of melon
3 oz/75 g offal (lambs' kidneys/chicken liver/lambs'
    liver) fried with ½ an onion
glass of fruit juice

Mid-morning
1 glass fruit juice

Lunch
4 oz/100 g minced meat with grated carrot and peas
    braised with onion, olive oil and vegetable stock
a selection of green vegetables lightly cooked
1 glass fruit juice

Mid-afternoon
2 glasses mineral water
1 whole fruit

Evening meal
lentil soup with carrots and celery (see recipes, page 259)
1 hard-boiled egg and 2 oz/50g prawns or shrimps
tasty salad (see recipes, page 269)

Bedtime
any amount of allowed hot drink

DAY 4

(Quick-serve lunch, pre-cooked evening meal)

On rising
2 glasses of mineral water

Breakfast
1 whole fruit
4 oz/100 g smoked haddock with 1 poached egg
1 glass of fruit juice

Mid-morning
1 glass of fruit juice

Lunch
6 oz/150 g gammon rasher (or other steak) fried in olive
    oil, topped with pineapple if desired
peas
green beans
carrots
1 glass fruit juice

Mid-afternoon
2 glasses mineral water
1 whole fruit

Evening meal
bowl of vegetable paste stock to drink with a spoon
bean salad (see recipes, page 272)
green salad: lettuce, cucumber and watercress
mineral water to drink with meal

Bedtime
any amount of allowed hot drink

DAY 5

(Easy-pack lunch, slow-cook evening meal)

On rising
2 glasses of mineral water

Breakfast
whole grapefruit
4 oz/100 g kippers poached in water
1 glass of fruit juice

Mid-morning
1 glass fruit juice

Lunch
4 oz/100 g chicken (cold or hot)
chewy salad (see recipe, page 268)
1 glass of fruit juice

Mid-afternoon
2 glasses mineral water
1 whole fruit

Evening meal

vegetable soup (at least 3 vegetables pureed in stock)
lamb chop braised in olive oil with celery and mush-
    rooms in a little vegetable stock
carrots and peas

Bedtime

any amount of allowed hot drink

DAY 6

(Easy-pack lunch, larger cooked evening meal)

On rising

2 glasses of mineral water

Breakfast

an orange and an apple chopped up together in a little
    lemon juice
sardines (in olive oil) hot or cold
1 glass of fruit juice

Mid-morning

1 glass fruit juice

Lunch

2 hard-boiled eggs
chewy salad (see recipe, page 268)
1 glass of fruit juice

Mid-afternoon

2 glasses mineral water
1 whole fruit

Evening meal

pork loin chop grilled
mixed vegetables (at least three) lightly cooked
banana

Bedtime
any amount of allowed hot drink

DAY 7

(Cooked lunch, quick-serve evening meal)

Breakfast
2 whole fruits chopped together in orange juice with
    2 tsps of sesame seeds sprinkled over
2 lambs' kidneys fried with half an onion
2 tbsps of pease pudding (see receipe, page 253)
1 glass of fruit juice

Mid-morning
1 glass fruit juice

Lunch
4 oz/100 g cooked beef
peas or green beans
carrots
1 whole fruit
1 glass of fruit juice

Mid-afternoon
2 glasses mineral water

Evening meal
bean salad (see recipe, page 272)
prawns or crab
lettuce
1 whole fruit

Bedtime
any amount of allowed hot drink

OPTION 3: CHANGING THE TIME THAT YOU EAT

This option can be used together with any of the first two options, while still following the plan. This option changes the way you take in your food so that the largest meal of the day is breakfast and the smallest is taken in the evening. Try eating a big breakfast, a medium-sized lunch, and a very light meal in the evening for a few weeks.

At the moment your evening meal is probably the biggest meal of the day, but what do you do afterwards? Nothing! Changing the time you eat will help you to lose weight, simply because you burn more calories in the daytime. I suggest that you try following the plan carefully while varying your meals in this way for three weeks, and see if you lose a few pounds. This could be the answer for people who do not have the time or inclination to follow complicated slimming diets, and the gradual weight loss can add up to a considerable amount over time.

You learned about the importance of breakfast in Chapter 3 (page 56) and the energy it gives you through the day, but to start eating a big breakfast suddenly can be very difficult. You can begin this new regime by not eating an evening meal at all one day: the next morning you will be really hungry for your breakfast! If you reduce your evening meal considerably from then on, you will gradually get into a new eating regime. This option suits me, as I wake up early in the morning really ready for my breakfast, and even though it takes a little longer to prepare and eat than usual, my hunger always gets me up in good time!

OPTION 4: FASTING

By the word 'fasting' I mean a short period when you drink plenty of clear fluids, but you do not eat. A short fast of one or two days is not harmful for most people, but fasting for longer than this is most inadvisable. If you are pregnant or unwell, do not fast deliberately.

If you are ill, fasting is nature's way of speeding recovery, and many people lose their appetite for a day or two with a bad cold, an infection or a severe stomach upset. In this case fasting seems to help recovery – if combined with plenty of rest. You can use short fasts to help your weight loss and general health, but always combine fasting with rest. If you are feeling really down, take a day of complete rest:

A special rest day for busy people

1. Drink as much as you like of: fresh water; fruit juices; mineral waters; herb teas; lemon juice sweetened with honey; black tea; black coffee; clear soup made from stock paste.

2. Eat nothing all day except: 1 apple; 1 orange; 1 pear.

3. Do nothing!

Don't go out.

Don't talk to anyone all day!

Take the phone off the hook.

Sleep as much as you can.

Words cannot describe how good it feels to do this: try to experience it for yourself at least once. It is a complete rest for the body, mind and spirit.

There are those who advocate a short fast as a regular practice, and you could accelerate your weight loss by doing this, but do not fast more than one day a week. Never exercise vigorously on a fast day: choose only gentle activity, if any, and make it a time of reflection and calm.

If you still tend to binge even while on the four zero plan, do not use the fast day as a way to punish yourself, or it may trigger another extended episode of bingeing and fasting. You will find more details about dealing with binges in Chapter 13.

OPTION 5: EXERCISE

This option can be used while following the plan and in conjunction with any of the other slimming options.

Do not exercise if you do not feel well enough. Leave it until you have the energy to enjoy it. Increasing your exercise can be an important part of losing weight. A fairly painless way is to try to have at least twenty minutes of continuous reasonably vigorous exercise every day. This could be a brisk one-mile walk with the dog, twenty minutes of scrubbing a floor, or washing windows, or try twenty minutes on an exercise bike. The trick is to do it *every day*, and preferably out of doors. The daylight will encourage your skin to top up your Vitamin D and the weight-bearing exercise will strengthen your bones.

The winners' walk: A simple exercise routine to get you fit

1. Walk for a continuous half-hour every day – turn round and come home after *exactly* fifteen minutes.

2. Take exactly the same route and try to walk a little faster each day.

3. Take note of the precise point you reach after *exactly* fifteen minutes on each walk, and see the distance from home increasing.

4. Change your route each week to avoid boredom.

5. Build a Winners' Walk into your lunch hour too on the same principle, and persuade a friend to join in the fun!

OPTION 6: ADAPTING ANOTHER DIET

Any other diet can be adapted to conform with the zero plan by using substitutes for any of the four zero foods mentioned in the menus, and most of the well-known calorie-controlled diets can be adapted to accord with the zero plan. The 'slim week' allows you about 1,300–1,700 calories a day, assuming moderate portions. One of the easiest ways to lose weight is to follow the basic plan, but keep your calorie intake to between 1,500 and 1,700 per day.

OPTION 7: SLIMMING GROUPS

There are a large number of slimming clubs operating nationwide. You may be able to follow a diet at your local club while still following the four zero plan.

Frances joins the club
This is how Frances described her experience of joining a local slimming club after the experiment:

'I have joined a slimming club and find their diet easier to follow now I have cut out all those little treats made from zero ingredients. it means that I can have more of other foods to make up the calorie allowance. I had tried the club's diet before, but it is much easier to follow this time.'

The no-grains option can easily be kept to about 1,500 calories a day and still be satisfying and healthy, so it accords very well with the low-calorie diets recommended by slimming clubs.

Winners' Groups
Start a Winners' Group. There are details of this on page 301.

CHAPTER 10
Tackling Other Addictions

So far in this book we have dealt only with the addiction to food. This chapter will deal with four other common addictions: alcohol, chocolate, caffeine and nicotine.

The object of this chapter is to help you to bring your addictions under control. In each case we will consider ways of reducing consumption but, as you discovered during the experiment, there is only one way to be completely free of your fix – and that is to give it up altogether. However, you may find with these much stronger addictions that it is better to be eased gently into giving up through a short period of reduced consumption, rather than moving from heavy consumption to total abstinence. For this reason you will find it helpful to remain on the four zero plan while you follow the advice in this chapter for, as you will see from the case histories, the four zero plan helps to reduce your consumption of alcohol, chocolate, caffeine and tobacco and makes a useful starting point for giving them up.

What's your poison?
Tick any of the following that you take in some form or other at least once every day:

alcoholic drinks	cola drinks
chocolate	painkillers with caffeine
cocoa	cigarettes
coffee	cigars
tea	tobacco

If you have ticked any one of the above, then you may need the advice in this chapter!

BEING AN ADDICT

By the term 'addict' I mean a person who takes some of their fix every day. This was the criterion used for food addiction and it will be continued here. Addiction exists on a sliding scale from a subtle, almost unnoticeable effect to a devastating and destructive influence. The potential for addiction lies all around us, and the substance we choose for a fix is really a matter of chance and availability, whether it's tobacco or toast, gambling or gâteau.

Every addiction develops along the same lines, through discovery of a source of satisfaction and pleasure, via increased consumption towards an inability to stop (see pages 84–5). The person concerned never admits to his addiction until the addiction itself becomes a problem.

AN ADDICTIVE PERSONALITY?

It is said that some people become addicts because they have an 'addictive personality', and change from one fix to another throughout life, never giving up their basic need for an addiction of some kind. This, surely, is not a personality problem, but a perfectly natural desire to seek pleasure and comfort wherever it can be found. I believe that, if there is such a thing as an 'addictive personality', it is just part of being human, and is probably something we all share.

THE ADDICTION PYRAMID

The addiction pyramid below will show you which addictions are the strongest. At the top is the addiction to 'hard' drugs, that ruins lives and kills hundreds of young people every year. At the bottom is food addiction; this can exert an influence for a lifetime but remain unnoticed by everyone, including you.

HEROIN
OTHER OPIATES
NATURAL DRUGS
SYNTHETIC DRUGS
CHEMICALS, GLUES, SOLVENTS
NICOTINE (cigarettes, tobacco)
ALCOHOL (wines, spirits, beers, lagers)
CAFFEINE (tea, coffee, cola drinks)
THEOBROMINE (chocolate, cocoa)
SUGARS (beet and cane sugar, fructose, honey)
WEAK ALKALOIDS (potato family)
STARCHES (grains, starch foods, root vegetables)
PROTEINS (meats, fish, milk protein, eggs, beans, seeds)
OILS AND FATS (vegetable oils, margarine, meat fat, butter)

(Freely adapted from Theron C. Randolph and Ralph Moss, *Allergies: Your Hidden Enemy* (Thorsons, 1984).)

FOOD-DRUG COMBINATIONS

If you become addicted to a food that is also a source of a drug, it can be hard to decide whether you are addicted to the drug or the food. We will consider the implications of this later in the relevant sections.

BEATING ADDICTIONS

Whether or not we remain addicted to our fix depends on a wide variety of factors, including our public attitude to addiction itself. While we continue to regard all addicts as weak-willed social outcasts, we are perpetuating a myth that makes it hard for anyone to admit to their own addictions.

161

STRESS AND ADDICTION

Stress can keep you addicted, because the more stress you have in your life, the more endorphins you will require to help you cope. When you are overtired, endorphins and adrenaline can keep you going, and at times like these the faster you gain satisfaction, the better. Alcohol, caffeine drinks and sugary foods can give you a lift almost at once, so people often use them to keep going under pressure.

In Chapter 5 we discussed the eight stages that everyone must go through to overcome any addiction. I have listed them below because it is useful to keep them in mind throughout this chapter:

1. Admission and awareness
2. Giving up
3. See an end to cravings
4. Gain rewards
5. Feeling deprived
6. Lapse and collapse
7. Feelings of control
8. Acceptance

Step one is to admit the addiction. By means of the four zero experiment you will have become aware of your tendency towards addiction, and now you are ready to tackle some of your other, stronger addictions by the same method.

ALCOHOL ADDICTION

When I use the term 'alcohol addict' I do not mean 'alcoholic'. What precisely is meant by alcoholism is outside the scope of this book, and is largely a matter of opinion. If you drink alcohol every day or several times a day, though, you are an alcohol addict according to the terms used here.

REDUCING ALCOHOL ON THE EXPERIMENT

You may have been surprised how much you reduced your intake when you drank only wine and cider during the experiment. One candidate thought that four pints of beer was a good drink in the evening, but was surprised to find that two pints of cider was more than enough for him! In fact, 36 per cent of candidates reduced their alcohol consumption during the trials, even though alcohol was allowed.

People naturally like alcoholic drinks for the stimulating and pleasant stress-relieving effects of the alcohol itself, but you may also develop a craving for the ingredients used to make it. Beer, lager and most spirits are made from a mixture of various grains, often including wheat. If you are a grain addict you may be attracted to beer for two reasons: the grains and the alcohol.

If you were unable to reduce your consumption of alcohol during the experiment, you may also be craving apples in cider or grapes in wine. Bear this in mind before you leap to the conclusion that alcohol alone is your problem.

ADDICTION TO ALCOHOL

If you simply cannot resist any kind of alcoholic drink, then alcohol is your fix and there is only one answer for you: total abstinence from all alcohol until your cravings have died enough to enable you to take an occasional drink and leave it at that.

WHY GIVE IT UP?

An excess of alcohol has no place on a slimming diet or a healthy-eating regime. Addiction to alcoholic drinks leads to overdose of alcohol itself, which puts a strain on the liver. The ingredients can trigger off food cravings. Alcohol itself can aggravate symptoms of food intolerance; it is a stimulant; and it can aggravate symptoms of anxiety or panic. Alcoholic drinks are high in calories and interfere with weight loss. An excess of alcohol deplete the body of B vitamins, and interfere with the metabolism of essential fatty acids.

GIVING IT UP

If you have a real problem with alcohol itself, a total ban is the only answer. Drink non-alcoholic beverages only, but do not use non-alcoholic beers – for you may be getting your fix from the grains in the beer rather than the alcohol. However, if you find that your consumption is reasonable if you avoid particular drinks, then you may be able to enjoy a drink from time to time – but *not* every day!

WITHDRAWAL

If you have been drinking alcohol on a regular basis, withdrawal symptoms can be quite severe following a total ban, e.g. headache, trembling hands and dizziness. If you moved to a different kind of alcohol on the experiment and still had withdrawal symptoms, then you are probably addicted to the ingredients of what was once your favourite tipple, and only you will know what that was! Withdrawal doesn't have to last for long if you keep to a healthy diet and give yourself plenty of other fluids, fresh air and gentle exercise.

PITFALLS

When you reach the deprivation stage (stage 5) do recognise this for what it is: your body still turning to alcohol to cope with a small crisis. Remember that this feeling too will pass if you keep going, taking one day at a time. The final stage is to accept that this problem is for life, and that you will always have to be careful not to slip into your alcohol habit again.

ALKALOIDS

On page 35 you were introduced to the *solanacae* plant family, of which the potato plant is a member. All the members of this family contain alkaloids of various kinds.

Alkaloids are chemicals that have an effect on the brain and nervous system. All alkaloids are highly addictive as they activate the same centres of the brain as our own endorphins and give us the same feelings of pleasure and satisfaction – but of course to varying degrees – and one alkaloid can easily be substituted for another.

If you treat the remaining nightshades as zero foods, this will reduce the total number of alkaloids in your diet and in turn reduce your cravings for the other sources of alkaloids in chocolate, caffeine drinks and tobacco. This was an effect widely experienced during the trials, when all the nightshades were banned from the beginning.

The remaining nightshades are tomatoes, all kinds of peppers and aubergines. Most of us in Britain can manage without aubergines very well, but peppers and tomatoes are hard to replace, particularly for lovers of Italian food.

TOMATOES

Tomatoes are found in almost every tin of soup and canned stew. They are also the base of many dishes and one of our children's favourite foods – baked beans. Children easily become hooked on the flavour of tomato ketchup and real addicts will refuse any savoury dish that does not have a dollop of tomato sauce upon it. 'Cream of tomato' is the biggest seller in every range of canned soups.

Living without tomatoes can be hard at first, but it can be done, believe me! For that strong flavour, use mushrooms, garlic, celery and onion in casseroles and salads.

For colour in salads use grated carrot, radish, beetroot and sweetcorn, or try the American habit of mixing vegetables with fruit.

PEPPERS

This group includes every kind of pepper you can imagine, except for the black and white pepper you grind over your food. Included in this list are the chillies in your hot sauce and the green and red peppers in your salad.

NIGHTSHADE-FREE FOR EVER?

One day when you have begun to control your addiction you will be able to bring back the nightshades again from time to time; but now you realise just how hooked you once were, don't let yourself slip into the tomato/pepper habit again.

CHOCOLATE ADDICTION

REDUCING CHOCOLATE DURING THE EXPERIMENT

As it is sugar-based, chocolate was banned during the experiment, but it was one of the principal reasons for later diet breakdown among candidates, with Easter being the main stumbling block.

Margaret (a milk and sugar addict) lost all her extra weight during the three-week experiment, and was heading confidently into the future with her new diet intact when Easter eggs came and put a stop to all that! The chocolate triggered off all her other cravings and she ate so much that in just a few weeks her weight was higher than ever before and she was in despair.

The cocoa powder in chocolate is addictive, being a source of theobromine (which is an alkaloid), but chocolate is a food-drug combination, and milk chocolate is made of cocoa, sugar and milk. Margaret, like many others, lost her desire for chocolate during the experiment because it was the sugar and milk she really craved. She soon realised this and was able to use the restart plan to begin again. The next year there were no chocolate eggs for Margaret, and she now knows how to come through Easter unscathed!

WHY GIVE IT UP?

Chocolate is handy, cheap, available from legal outlets almost twenty-four hours a day, and socially acceptable. It tastes good and has no immediate side-effects. Add to this the image, convenience, eatability and 'naughtiness' factor of chocolate, and you have a very versatile and delicious fix indeed!

The dangers of eating too much chocolate lie in the space it takes up in the diet. It is so easy to snack off chocolate, or even dine off it. There is only so much room in your stomach and your day for eating, and while you are eating chocolate you are not eating real, fresh, whole food to keep you healthy.

While a chocolate addiction is at work, there is little possibility of permanent weight loss, for chocolate is high in calories. Chocolate consumption is related to migraines and, as the theobromine is a stimulant, it can induce feelings of edginess or even panic. Chocolate is a favourite binge food, and is best avoided completely in order to starve cravings for it.

GIVING IT UP

During the experiment chocolate was banned as it contains sugar, and often milk. You probably lost your taste for it quite quickly in the first week, and as long as you avoid it completely for a considerable time, you will soon be free of your cravings for it.

Useful substitutes for chocolate sweets are dried fruits such as dates or figs. Carob powder can be used in recipes instead of cocoa.

WITHDRAWAL

A confirmed chocoholic can feel quite ill when her chocolate is banned. Usual symptoms are headaches, insomnia and an overwhelming sense of fatigue. When you give up chocolate you must make sure that you eat a good healthy diet, rich in raw foods to help you to readjust to a chocolate-free diet. As it is based on whole, fresh food, the Food Addict's Diet is ideal for this purpose, and every one of the chocolate addicts trying the experiment found that their withdrawal symptoms had passed completely by the end of the first week.

PITFALLS

Many people feel a strong craving for other sweet things to replace chocolate, and this illustrates how the sugar element plays an important part in their chocolate addiction.

If you find yourself in an impossible or frustrating situation then you will experience that feeling of deprivation and go in search of chocolate. Remember that at times of stress we all feel the need for a fix, but it does nothing to remove the stress! Offering someone chocolate when they are under stress is like offering a man a cigarette in the desert instead of a drink: he may feel better, but he is still thirsty. Whatever happens, always remember the restart plan is there to pick you up again if you do give in.

CAFFEINE DRINKS

CAFFEINE DRINKS AND THE FOUR ZERO EXPERIMENT

On the trials about half of the candidates found their consumption of caffeine drinks increasing during the experiment, but by the end of the experiment 52 per cent of candidates had reduced their consumption of tea and coffee, and 21 per cent of those had given it up altogether! Why were there two such contradictory effects?

The candidates who could drink their tea and coffee black kept up their habit, but the rest could not enjoy it without milk and gave it up with little difficulty. Tea and coffee with milk and sugar is a food-drug combination, and clearly one group was craving the milk and possibly the sugar too, and the other group needed the caffeine. A common reason for refusing to take part in the experiment was having to drink tea without milk, and this group presumably were addicted to the milk as much as the tea.

ADDICTION TO CAFFEINE

Caffeine is the world's favourite drug, and you can be a caffeine 'junkie' without knowing it. Caffeine is to be found in tea, coffee and cola drinks. The greatest concentration is found in strong coffee, which will give you 100 mg of caffeine per cup. A cup of strong tea will give you 50 mg, so just moving from coffee to tea will halve your caffeine intake. Cola drinks are relatively low in caffeine and it is possible to get caffeine-free cola these days. Taking more than 250 mg of caffeine at a time is likely to have a significant physical effect upon you. This amount would be obtained from either three cups of strong coffee, four cups of tea, or seven cans of cola.[1]

WHY GIVE IT UP?

People vary according to how sensitive they are to caffeine, and some people will feel the effects of even one cup of tea almost at once, and will even react to decaffeinated coffee. Effects of too much caffeine include a rapid pulse, anxiety, nervousness, insomnia, the 'restless legs' syndrome, panic attacks, abnormal heart rhythms, tremor and migraine.[2] Some pain killers contain caffeine (e.g. Anadin), so be careful to cut these out also.

As caffeine stimulates gastric secretion, it can also cause acid indigestion. The tannin in tea prevents the absorption of iron and zinc from food, and contributes to anaemia. People with a tendency to anaemia should therefore be careful not to drink too many cups of tea, and especially not with food. Also, women who suffer from lumpy breasts and breast pain may find an improvement after giving up caffeine drinks; so if that is your problem, try it, even if you believe that you are not hooked on caffeine at all.[3]

GIVING IT UP

First of all, go and buy decaffeinated coffee and tea, but remember that the tiny amount of caffeine that remains will be enough to keep your cravings alive, so aim to remove this too. For substitutes try herb teas, additive-free stock cubes or Vecon paste (obtainable from good supermarkets or health-food stores), dandelion coffee, and so on, but be careful of some ersatz coffees if you are on a grain-free diet. Buy a box of mixed herbal tea bags to help you to discover your favourites. Remember that only complete elimination of caffeine will kill your cravings for it. Aim eventually to cut out tea, coffee, cocoa and cola drinks (even those with only tiny amounts of caffeine) from your diet completely.

WITHDRAWAL

Caffeine is such a strong drug that you will possibly get a withdrawal headache in the first two days or feel sleepy and lethargic. If you do have withdrawal symptoms, remember that this is a sign that your body is heaving a sigh of relief, so welcome them!

PITFALLS

There is very strong social pressure on us to drink coffee and tea. If you are already a known tea drinker, it is a little embarrassing to have to explain how you have given it up. The simplest thing to ask for is a cup of plain hot boiled water in the winter, or a cold drink in summer. Decaffeinated coffee is becoming increasingly common in restaurants, etc., and is a useful substitute in the absence of anything else, but take care: if you are a real caffeine addict, you may find that just one cup of tea or coffee will trigger off your addictive cravings again.

NICOTINE

REDUCING NICOTINE ON THE EXPERIMENT

As you live with the zero plan, month after month, you will begin to feel calmer, and cope better with stress. This will mean that your psychological need for cigarettes will decline. Once all the nightshades, tea, coffee and chocolate are avoided, the physical effects of each cigarette will seem that much stronger and more satisfying. Therefore, fewer cigarettes are required to have the same effect. Without tiny doses of any kind of alkaloid to keep those cravings alive, they will quietly die of starvation and giving up will be that much easier.

Jane, one of my earliest guinea pigs, decided to give up smoking altogether after six months of following the plan, and found it remarkably easy. She had given up many times before but this time she has not yet yielded to the temptation to start smoking again, which surprises her. She is careful not to take any caffeine drinks or nightshades in case her cravings are triggered off again.

ADDICTION TO NICOTINE

Nicotine is the drug in tobacco and it is an alkaloid. The harmful effects of tobacco have been documented *ad nauseam*, and I will not repeat it all here.

If you are trying to help someone to give up, do not be afraid to tell them that you prefer them not to smoke in your house. Peer pressure can be used as a potent force in both causing and preventing addictions, so let's use it to reduce the number of places where smokers can smoke. Not only will this reduce the effects on the rest of us, but people trying to give up will be helped by not being sub- jected to the tempting sight of a smoking cigarette every- where they go.

GIVING IT UP

If you smoke already, don't say you cannot give up. You can if you decide to. Remember Tony on page 84? Hun- dreds of people kick the smoking habit every day, and so can you. Just take those eight steps to overcoming addic- tion one by one, and you will do it.

WITHDRAWAL

As cigarette smoke damages your lungs and throat, with- drawal symptoms can sometimes be outweighed by the disappearance of a cough, a husky voice and the stale taste in your mouth. However, you can suffer headache, irri- tability, fatigue and even vomiting as withdrawal symp- toms. Remember that withdrawal is a sign of the poisons leaving your body and represents an important step towards being free of a dirty and very dangerous habit.

PITFALLS

The usual pitfall is thinking that you will cope better with stress if you have 'just one', and that 'just one will not hurt'. In fact, you are kidding yourself. The tobacco will do nothing to save the situation, and you know that. Just like the chocoholic, you think that you will cope better after a fix. In reality, you will cope less well, because your addictive cravings will return and you will have two problems to deal with!

You have taken one? Well, before the addiction grabs you, go back to page one, stage one: five days without a smoke and you will be over the worst cravings.

AN END TO ADDICTION?

At the beginning of this chapter we defined an addict as someone who needed his fix every day. You may have disagreed with this definition, but I hope you have found the advice helpful in surmounting any problem you have controlling the alcohol, caffeine drinks, chocolate and tobacco in your life.

If you were not an addict you would be happy to take just a little tea, one piece of chocolate and perhaps an occasional cigarette once or twice a week and not look for any more. Perhaps one day you may be able to control your cravings enough to do this and enjoy 'just a little' knowing that at last a little need not become a lot: then you will have won your addiction battle.

CHAPTER 11
Coping with Food Intolerance

The true causes of food intolerance are far from clear, and are unfortunately too complex to include in a book of this kind. If you would like to find out more about how food intolerance symptoms arise, read Dr John Brostoff's *Food Allergy and Intolerance* (Bloomsbury, 1989). This is a readable account drawn from a formidable amount of experience of treating thousands of food-sensitive people.

In Chapter 2, you were introduced to a list of symptoms that usually resist all forms of treatment, sometimes fade and flare up again, and occur more frequently under stress: these are the symptoms of food intolerance.

FINDING THE CULPRIT

Isolating the food that is causing the trouble is much like detective work. A food will not cause symptoms unless it is eaten frequently, so your suspect will be one of the food ingredients you eat most often. Your food diary (see pages 75–6) will have already indicated these. The four zero foods were selected as being by far the most likely suspects, but there may be more, and this chapter will show you how to find them.

TEST AND REST

An elimination diet is both a test to tell you which foods are the cause of the problem, and a rest to relieve you of your symptoms. To begin an elimination diet you choose a food and eliminate it from your diet completely. If you have been reacting to it, this will give your body a complete rest from it. Then, once your body is no longer being bombarded by an excessive amount of a substance it can't cope with, you will see an improvement in your symptoms – after the initial period of withdrawal.

However, if you eat the culprit food again once your body has fully readjusted to being without it, you may experience a noticeable reaction. This is because your body is no longer adapted to having the food constantly present, and is 'surprised' into a reaction. This unexpected reaction to a food you once could eat with impunity is a clear indication of food intolerance, and is a useful test for it.

FOUR OTHER FACTORS IN FOOD INTOLERANCE

If you can establish a definite relationship between eating a food and a flare-up in your symptoms, then you will have definitely isolated the culprit. This may seem quite simple and clear-cut explained in this way, but in practice there is rarely any clear link between exactly what you have eaten and how you now feel: there are several other factors to be taken into account when trying to explain why your symptoms flare and fade.

INHERITANCE

Perhaps your mother has asthma when she eats oranges, and you have migraine when you eat chocolate; in that case, you have not inherited your mother's asthma, but you have inherited the basic tendency to react, which can produce a wide range of symptoms, both physical and mental, throughout the family.

STRESS

Symptoms occur more frequently when you are under stress, and are more frequent during or immediately after long periods of stress or illness. Intolerance symptoms can be triggered by the stresses of major hormone change, such as puberty, pregnancy and the menopause, or even the prolonged use of steroid drugs such as the contraceptive pill.

HEALTH

If you are generally run down, exhausted or badly nourished, you will be less tolerant of your food.

OVERDOSE

We all tend to become sated or bored when constantly exposed to the same thing, and this applies as much to food as to anything else. Your body was designed for fine tuning, and not for coping with overdose, and too much of any food ingredient taken at once can overwhelm your ability to cope.

OVERLOAD

If you have a tendency to react in any case, are under stress and run down, and exposed just once too often to a particular food ingredient, then you will know moments or even longer periods of 'overload', when your symptoms will be at their worst.

EASING THE LOAD

To ease your symptoms you need not enter into the rather confusing business of isolating culprit foods. The first and most important step is to reduce the stresses in your life as far as you can and learn to cope with those stresses you cannot avoid. Always try to avoid as far as you can those moments of overload when you are asking too much of your body: give yourself plenty of rest and quiet when you need it.

The second step is to eat wholesome food in the greatest variety you can afford, and not expose your system to any substances that you already know cause a reaction. In the preceding chapters there has been a great deal of advice to help you to do this, as well as the four zero plan to cut out the four most important culprits and bring that all-important variety back into your diet.

The third step is to build up your general health with vitamin and mineral supplements, particularly zinc, which boosts your immune system and is generally deficient in the British diet. (Zinc-rich foods allowed on the four zero plan are wholegrains other than wheat, and seeds, nuts and meats.)

Ideally, the final step would be to remove from your life all the substances that affect you, but unfortunately that is not possible. Any number of substances other than food, such as chemicals in the air we breathe, can aggravate your food intolerance symptoms by increasing the load on your body. The best we can hope for is to reduce the load wherever possible while building up your ability to cope with it by improving your health.

THE SUSPECTS

If the four zero plan and the lifestyle changes it has already created have not brought you a sufficient improvement in your symptoms, this section will show you how to draw up a list of your personal suspect foods and test them to see if they are playing a part in your problem.

NOTE: Another, rather more expensive, way to draw up your list of personal suspects is to take a food allergy/ intolerance test. There are a variety of different tests available, based on many different theories, and a test can be a useful way to discover your suspects. Once you have your list of culprits, you can eliminate them all at once, or one by one as a test (see page 184).

TEN GROUPS OF SUSPECTS

From the various books I have read and from my experiences on the trials, I have put together a list of the substances (foods, drinks, drugs) that are most likely to be the causes of your food intolerance symptoms. By working our way through this list we will come up with a list of your personal suspects, and eliminate them one by one until we have created the perfect diet for you.

The major pointer to each of the suspects will be signs of addiction, for if you are addicted to a substance you will tend to overdose on it, and the overdose aggravates the symptoms, as we have seen on page 176; so to create your list of suspects, make a note of any of those items mentioned below that you take every day.

NOTE: You will notice that there are several other foods that could have been included in groups 3–10. I have left them out and included only the most commonly eaten members of each group.

Group 1: the other nightshades (see Chapter 10)

These are tomatoes, peppers and aubergines, and we looked at them in detail in Chapter 10. I hope that, if alkaloids are your problem, they have already become three extra zeros.

Group 2: non-foods (see Chapter 10)

Tea, coffee and cigarettes
When you have succeeded in conquering your addictions, at least for a while, with the help of Chapter 10, see if there is any improvement in your symptoms. If so, it may not be necessary for you to go any further down this list.

Alcohol
Red wine is not allowed on the plan as it is often cited as a suspect in food intolerance, possibly because it has several chemical additives that are not present in white wines. Many more people react to red wine than white, and that is why it is banned during the experiment. If you have missed your red wine a great deal during the experiment, and have been tempted time and again to drink some, you have found another suspect – for your dependence on it is a sure sign that you are reacting to it (see Martin's case study, pages 230–2).

Your addictions could be a useful pointer to the problem here: if you find that you are drinking white wine or cider every single day, you are addicted either to the alcohol or the ingredients, which are yeast, apples or grapes. If you react to yeast you will probably also show a yen for Marmite and other yeast extracts, and if you react to apples you will probably love apple juice most of all the fruit juices, and prefer cider to wine. If you react to grapes, then you will also be a lover of fruit cakes and mincemeat as well as wine and fresh grapes.

Food additives
Artificial additives should have almost left your diet by now, because processed foods so often contain the four zero foods and are therefore not allowed on the diet. Avoid any allowed foods with artificial additives as far as possible and concentrate on real, whole, fresh food. Do this whether you think food additives are your

problem or not, and as soon as possible, for the fewer chemicals your body has to deal with, the better.

Chemicals in your house

What chemicals are there in your life? Perhaps you think you do not use any at all, but look in the kitchen, the bedroom, the bathroom and the garden shed. Any of these chemicals, splashed or sprayed around, can cause symptoms in sensitive individuals. Richard Mackarness's book, *Chemical Victims* (Pan, 1980), deals with the role of chemicals in illnesses of various kinds, both physical and mental.

Try biodegradable chemical products: not only are they environmentally friendly, but they are people friendly too! Ventilate your house by opening the windows and doors for at least half an hour each day – rain or shine – and this will prevent the build-up of fumes and vapours from your furniture, paint or gas fire. Use cosmetics and personal products that are free from perfumes and other additives, including soap, shower gel, deodorant and make-up. Remember that any small step you can take to reduce overload will also reduce your symptoms.

When you come to test this group, you will have great difficulty avoiding every single chemical, so don't even try. Just do what you can to cut the chemicals you use to a minimum. You will find it remarkably easy, and not expensive: just avoid all unnecessary cleaning fluids and deodorising sprays and use fresh air and elbow grease instead!

Chemicals on your food

Theron Randolph and Ralph Moss's book, *Allergies: Your Hidden Enemy* (Thorsons, 1984), strongly suggests that many so-called food intolerance reactions could well be reactions to chemical residues left on foods, from insecticides and fungicides sprayed on to growing plants or stored food. For example, someone who was unable to eat apples without getting symptoms

might be able to eat apples grown without chemicals –
perhaps from a long-neglected orchard – with impunity.
So, before you embroil yourself in the tangle of trying
to establish which food makes you react, consider a
week or two on nothing but organically grown foods,
and see how well you feel when you are freed from
those chemical residues: you may be in for a pleasant
surprise!

Group 3: four other grains (see Chapter 9)

These are barley, oats, rye and corn. If you do not need
to lose weight you may not have tried the grain-free diet
on pages 144–7, which eliminates all four of these, so
I suggest you read it carefully before testing these
suspects.

Corn

If you live in the United States and are of American
origin, then you have probably eaten corn every day of
your life. It is very likely that you are intolerant and
addicted to it. In that case, make corn a fifth zero.

Rice: a useful substitute

Notice that rice has not been included in this group.
Intolerance to rice is very rare in Britain, and is generally found only in those countries where they eat it
almost to the exclusion of everything else. You can use
rice boiled or fried in place of potatoes, rice cakes in
place of bread, and flaked rice in place of porridge oats.

   The other starchy foods that can be used as often as
you wish are: millet, buckwheat, sago, tapioca and
arrowroot.

Group 4: soya

Soya beans and milk, tofu and miso have probably
found their way into your diet recently in far greater
quantities than before, mainly as substitutes for the
four zeros. Soya is a concentrated protein food, and
many people are sensitive to it.

Soya is the principal suspect food in Japan, so if you are of Japanese origin, make soya your fifth zero food.

Substitutes
In place of soya milk, use nut or seed milks (see recipes, pages 245–6). Anchovy sauce or vinaigrette dressing make a useful substitute for soy sauce; other beans can be used instead of soya beans; and garlic or mushroom paste (available from good supermarkets) tastes as good as miso in soup.

Group 5: peanuts
These are not in fact nuts, but legumes. Peanuts are grown in America and Australia, and feature strongly in the diet of these countries. Here in Britain we are fast developing a peanut habit, and as they are delicious raw with raisins they rapidly take a front seat as a snack for people on the four zero plan.

Substitutes
For nibbles, try seed mixes or chopped tropical fruits and seeds. In place of peanut butter, try tahini or sunflower paste, or make a nut butter with another nut (see recipe, page 250).

Group 6: other animal milks
If you have been substituting sheep's or goats' milk for cows' milk, these could also be culprits; for if you found that cows' milk aggravated any of your symptoms, you are highly likely to react to the other milks too. Sheep's milk is less often a culprit, so you may be able to get away with a little cheese or yoghurt made with sheep's milk.

Group 7: nuts
Nuts tend to become an important snack food to replace potato or wheat snacks on the four zero plan. Ready-shelled nuts are more likely to cause reactions, owing to fungicides used upon them to

prevent deterioration, so try to eat all your nuts straight from the shell.

Substitutes

Seeds (e.g. sunflower, pumpkin, sesame) can be mixed with a few dried fruits for a delicious snack, added to salads, and sprinkled over sweet foods.

Other less usual nuts (see list on page 101) are useful if, after the test, you are still not sure if you react to nuts or not. In this case, avoid your usual nuts and try some different ones.

Group 8: red meat

This means beef, lamb and pork. A few weeks without red meat can be an interesting experience for anyone, especially for people of North American origin, because beef in particular is eaten so frequently.

Beef and pork are 'factory farmed' and growth hormone is used to promote muscle. In theory, these hormones are given time to clear the system before slaughter; however, the fact that pork and beef are implicated in food intolerance more often than lamb may be related to the hormone treatment in some way.

Substitutes

There are plenty of other animals and birds to choose from for your meat (see list on page 100). However, a reduction in animal protein and saturated fat in your diet is good for you in any case, so try a vegetarian diet for a while and see if it suits you.

Group 9: eggs

There are only three kinds of egg to test: chicken, goose and duck. If you find you do react to chickens' eggs but have no reaction to other eggs, that will be a useful discovery.

Substitutes

There are other protein foods to choose from even if you are a vegetarian (beans, nuts, seeds, wholegrains), so if

183

you have become dependent on eggs for protein you had better get out of that rut!

Group 10: citrus fruits

This group consists of the more usual citrus fruits, including lemons, grapefruit, tangerines and satsumas. Intolerance to orange is common, particularly among children. The peel seems to be the main problem: sensitive people may be affected by citral, a natural chemical found in the peel of oranges and an antagonist to Vitamin A. Others may be reacting to residues of chemical sprays on the peel. Orange squash is made from both juice and peel, ground to a pulp and sweetened.

Any other fruit or fruit drink can be used as a substitute.

TESTING TIMES

The test is a three-step process, and it takes a month to test each suspect. First, you avoid the suspect group for two weeks, then you reintroduce the suspect alone for one week, and thirdly you introduce the other foods in the suspect group. These three steps can be repeated for each suspect. To make the test as easy as possible for you, here is a simple system for scoring symptoms, control and hunger.

A SCORING SYSTEM

Here is a scoring system to use on the testing form on page 186.

Symptoms	score
worse	1
the same	2
a little better	3
very much better	4
completely disappeared	5

184

Control over consumption of substance being tested

	score
no control at all	1
very poor control	2
poor control	3
quite good control	4
good control	5

General hunger	score
very hungry all the time	1
very hungry most of the time	2
quite hungry most of the time	3
only hungry at mealtimes	4
not very hungry at all	5

THE TEST

Test the suspect foods in order of your addiction to them, beginning with the suspects you eat most often and find hardest to resist.

Step 1: Avoiding the suspect group

See which food group your chosen suspect belongs to and avoid all the foods listed for that group. For example, if you find that you are taking goats' milk or cheese every day then avoid all of group 6 (goats' and sheep's milk) for two weeks, but do *not* mark the testing form yet.

Live without that whole group of foods for two weeks, and *at the end of the two weeks* make a note of your control over the suspect food, your hunger generally, your measurements and the state of your symptoms on the testing form in the 'before' column.

TESTING FORM

(This form can be copied or photocopied to test for other foods.)

Food being tested ....
From suspect group no ....

Control over consumption of food being tested

	Before	After
Score:	.....	.....

General hunger

	Before	After
Score:	.....	.....

Measurements	Before	After
Weight ... st ... lbs (..... kg)	.....	.....
Bust/chest ... in ... cm	.....	.....
Waist ... in ... cm	.....	.....
Hips ... in ... cm	.....	.....
Thighs (about 9" above knee)		
right ... in ... cm	.....	.....
left ... in ... cm	.....	.....
Upper arms		
right ... in ... cm	.....	.....
left ... in ... cm	.....	.....
Other ... in ... cm	.....	.....

NOTE: Sometimes a reaction shows as a swelling in another part of your body such as your ankles: if so, take these measurements too and note them down as 'other'.

Symptoms

My minor symptoms are:	Score before	Score after
a	....	....
b	....	....
c	....	....

d ....
e ....

New symptoms appearing when food is tested
a ....
b ....

NOTE: Your reaction to the food you are testing may not be a flare-up of your normal symptoms, but may take the form of completely new symptoms.

Step 2: Reintroducing the suspect food

During the two suspect-free weeks, there may have been a change for the better, but the real test of food intolerance comes when you eat the food again after your body has readjusted to living without it for some time. So for another week, start to eat the suspect food every day but do not eat any of the other foods in that particular group. The first time you take the food again, you may notice some kind of physical or mental reaction up to twelve hours after eating it. Note this carefully on the testing form. *At the end of the week* make a note of your new scores in the 'after' column on the testing form on page 186. If there are changes for the worst between the 'before' and 'after' scores, then avoid eating the food.

Step 3: Testing the other foods in the group

Reintroduce the rest of the group of foods the following week. If there is no further change in any of your scores, these foods are all safe to eat. If you have any further 'suspects' in this group, test them individually later. If you carry out these three steps on all the foods you eat most often, you will have created a new diet, tailor-made for you.

187

CHAPTER 12
Mainly for Women

There is much that women can do to take better care of themselves, and this chapter will show you how a change in your diet can help you to avoid some of the ill health that arises from the simple fact that you are female.

Being a woman is a major health risk, a fact that seems to be largely misunderstood, particularly by men. The biological status of women demands that they carry most of the stresses of family life, and simply to function as women they have to undergo a series of painful, life-threatening and debilitating experiences: pregnancy and childbirth, menstruation, and the hormone changes of late middle age.

MONTHLY MISERY

In modern industrial societies menstruation begins at about twelve years old and continues for another thirty-five years. In a lifetime a woman will experience about 480 menstrual cycles. Women stop menstruating if they become very thin, are under continuous physical or emotional stress, or if they stop ovulating.

A woman's experience of menstruation is often more than mere inconvenience and feeling mildly unwell. Menstruation often causes extreme fatigue, dizziness, fainting, stomach cramps, headaches, and a loss of libido. It occurs several hundred times in a woman's lifetime regardless of what other demands are being made upon her. Exams, performances, demanding work and family problems must all be tackled, despite the fact that for approximately a week every month she is not at her best.

All this comes after developing symptoms of pre-menstrual tension (PMT): irritability, depression, a craving for sweet food or alcohol, and mood swings. The symptoms of premenstrual tension are very similar to those minor symptoms listed on pages 41-3, and women who suffer from food intolerance find their symptoms get worse during their premenstrual week. There can be mental effects too: crime among women, and even suicide, has been associated with premenstrual tension.

These changes during the menstrual cycle are a real problem and a cause of great unhappiness for many women. It is a small wonder that women are regarded as fickle, neurotic, unreliable or weak: they must seem so! Unfortunately menstruation is often still a taboo subject – which is a shame, because it would save many problems if it were spoken about more openly.

APPETITE CHANGES DURING THE MONTH

During the first two weeks of the menstrual cycle, fol-lowing the onset of a period, compulsive eaters often gain a day or two of relief from their cravings, slimmers feel that at last they have things under control, and healthy appetites are aimed towards healthy, fresh, raw foods.

On or around the fourteenth day, ovulation creates a 'mini-PMT' episode that may last only a day, but can trigger off a longer bad-eating episode. We all know what such a bad-eating episode can do: all those foods you are addicted to suddenly become quite irresistible. Your diet intentions break down after only two weeks and there is an increase in weight. Seeing an increase in weight or just generally feeling low, even for a day, can bring about the guilt-eating cycle of diet breakdown.

In the week before your period is due, be ready for your PMT symptoms, such as bloating or weight gain. Notice an increased craving for sweet, starchy foods (for wheat and sugar, in fact). Once bleeding begins, you will be transformed from a ravenous biscuit-hunter into a slightly listless person who does not feel hungry – amazing!

PMT AND THE ZERO PLAN

The four zero plan and the grain-free option (see pages 144–7) are particularly helpful in relieving the symptoms of premenstrual tension.

You will find on the plan that your addictive cravings increase markedly in the premenstrual week; keep off all traces of the foods you crave, even if it means snacking ten times a day on allowed foods! In time you will find that the premenstrual week is easy to navigate, and you will emerge into daylight into another month without breaking your slimming diet or giving in to your addictions. Once you have broken this four-week barrier to your diet intentions, you will make excellent progress!

If you are slimming, make the premenstrual week grain-free, and once you have rediscovered your equilibrium, begin the 'slim week' (see page 147). The remaining weeks can be spent on the basic four zero plan as a diet rest.

Carla beats PMT with the Food Addict's Diet
Here is what Carla had to say about her experiences on the zero plan. She was a forty-two-year-old nurse, who needed to lose two stones in weight. However, she discovered another important benefit after about seven weeks: the zero plan cured her premenstrual tension:

'During premenstrual times and under stress I usually eat too much. My stomach swells up and I feel fat and ugly. Nothing fits properly. I find digestive biscuits quite irresistible in the two days before my period starts and things rise to a kind of crescendo the night before: I start to eat quantities of sweet stuff, I scream at everybody, hate the world and everything in it, including myself. I feel ashamed of my fat middle and of my lack of will power.

'Three days later I am calm and not at all hungry, but of course a great deal heavier owing to the overeating a few days before. This is a kind of merry-go-round that I can't get off. I can't stay on a slimming diet long enough to actually get anywhere!

'My first period on the plan was late and very scanty but I was not as irritable as usual, even though I broke the rules really badly the evening before! The next time I had a period was after two weeks being grain-free. Not only did I not have any of my usual premenstrual symptoms that time (i.e. weight gain, tiredness, irritability and abdominal pain), I did not even realise I had started! This period was on time, generally trouble-free and hardly more than a three-day hiccough in the month: bliss!'

We had already established that Carla had a grain sensitivity, and it is interesting to observe that while the four zero plan helped a little during the experiment, the grain-free fortnight helped much more. This seems to indicate a relationship between PMT and Carla's intolerance to food. She proved this later when she gave up the zero plan for two or three months and saw a return of all her old PMT symptoms when wheat and other grains were reintroduced into her diet.

MENOPAUSE: THE END TO MONTHLY MISERY?

Many women do not realise that even after the menopause the menstrual clock may still function, and the monthly 'alarm' may still go off from time to time. After

191

the menopause women are at last free of monthly bleeding, but unfortunately many of them still suffer occasional symptoms similar to PMT, such as mood swings or irritability. Many women notice regular mood swings and weight changes after the menopause, but once they have lost the yardstick of the monthly bleeding they do not relate these changes to a monthly cycle. Faced with inexplicable episodes of feeling emotional, extra hungry and tired, they are less able to cope than they might be if they realised what was happening.

If you have occasional bad attacks of any of your minor symptoms, make a note of the date when they are really severe. Mark your calendar with your bad days and after three or four months you will see a pattern emerging. Expect your appetite to get out of control once a month or so: if you predict it, you can cope with it.

Now that you have tried the experiment you may have already noticed that your hot flushes, fluid retention, headaches and lassitude have eased or completely disappeared. The symptoms of the menopause are very similar to food intolerance symptoms, and they may in fact be simply these, triggered off by the stress of those hormone changes.

PREGNANCY ON THE PLAN

Persistent headaches or vomiting, faintness or a constant feeling of nausea, agitation, extreme nervousness, fatigue or irritability in early pregnancy may be directly food-related. During pregnancy there is an increased requirement for calcium, and many women drink more milk than usual at this time. If you have an intolerance to milk you could develop symptoms of food intolerance during pregnancy due to an overdose of milk. The first four months of pregnancy are a time of hormone changes and you are more likely to show symptoms of food intolerance at this time.

The zero plan is safe to use while you are pregnant,

providing you take a calcium supplement to replace the calcium supply once obtained from milk. (See the Calci-Counter, on page 286.) Try three weeks on the zero plan and see if you feel any better. If you do, then your food may be to blame!

If you are still suffering, do not restrict your diet too much while you are pregnant by attempting any further eliminations. The best way to reduce your symptoms is to eat as much variety as possible with plenty of real, whole, raw food. Vary the ingredients of your diet from day to day to prevent overdosing on any single food. In this way, you can reduce the load on your body while you are carrying the baby. When the baby is born and you have recovered from the birth, then you can try the food tests on pages 184-7 to find the cause of any symptoms that may still persist.

BREASTFEEDING ON THE PLAN

If you have been following the zero plan during pregnancy, there is no need to stop in order to take cows' milk for calcium while you are breastfeeding, for it is not true that 'milk makes milk'. Your breasts are there to make milk, and they will, if you provide the right conditions. You will need to drink at least two litres of fluid a day while you are feeding, and eat a very rich, varied diet. The Food Addict's Diet will give you all the goodness you need to make good milk, provided you continue to take the calcium supplement.

You also need plenty of rest, both in mind and body. Successful breastfeeding is comforting in itself, and the hormones that help the milk secretion act like a kind of sedative: don't fight it! Just complete your normal basic domestic tasks, take as much time as possible off work, never feed baby in a hurry – and all will be well.

If you know you are intolerant to food, avoid the food that affects you and stop drinking tea, coffee and alcohol while you are breastfeeding. Colic and food intolerance symptoms in babies can be caused by the mother overdosing on a food and then feeding her baby milk that is loaded with molecules of the undigested food. These can pass into the baby's stomach and create food intolerance without the baby ever eating the food!

If you are breastfeeding and your baby has colic, try the four zero plan for a week or two and see if there is any improvement in your baby's general happiness. If he is less restless while you are on the plan, you may have been handing on your food intolerances to him through your breastmilk. You can find out more about dealing with colic in babies in Maureen Minchin's book, *Food for Thought* (OUP, 1984). This book is an interesting study that relates colic in babies to food intolerance, not only in the baby himself but the mother as well!

POSTNATAL DEPRESSION

Postnatal depression, being persistently overweight, and the onset of symptoms of food intolerance can all follow a pregnancy. Usually it is not the first pregnancy that causes the problem, but a subsequent one. Pregnancy, with the aftermath of huge hormone readjustments and the stress of coping with a new family member, can be a very traumatic experience indeed.

We tend to underestimate the long-term effect that the trauma of childbirth can have on a woman's health. During pregnancy there is a huge demand for vital nutrients, particularly calcium, zinc, iron, magnesium and the B vitamins. A very rich, varied diet is what is needed.

Women need as much physical and emotional support as possible from fathers to keep postnatal depression at bay. This is much better than tranquillisers – which can be addictive and create problems of their own later.

The stress and exhaustion of looking after a new baby can send a mother looking for comfort from her food. Even if she has managed to avoid gaining too much weight during pregnancy, she will gain weight now if she allows her addictive cravings full rein. The weight gain can add to feelings of depression and worthlessness. The four zero plan is an excellent way to prevent addictions arising at this time, and will provide all the healthy food you need for a speedy recovery without gaining weight.

After pregnancy there may be nutritional deficiencies caused by the enormous demands pregnancy and childbirth make on your body. These deficiencies can have marked effects on your mood and may aggravate postnatal depression. Deficiencies should be met by your deficiency cravings, but they will remain unnoticed and unanswered for months if your addictive cravings overwhelm them.

A very varied, healthy diet such as the Food Addict's Diet will establish a more natural pattern of nutrient supply and demand than simply supplementing the diet with vitamin pills – although these can be useful as an added benefit.

LAST IN THE FOOD LINE

Women have always put themselves last in the food line, when they should be first. They eat a far less healthy diet than they need to function well. All that is really required is a change of attitude: to believe that it is right for the woman to receive as much good food as the man – and sometimes more.

Women have the role of choosing and preparing food for others, but they can find it hard to think of what they need themselves. The Food Addict's Diet can help here.

Jean

Jean, who is a widow and who tried the experiment to lose weight, told me that she could never think of what to eat before she started the four zero plan. She used to ask her husband what he fancied, and eat the same food as him, but since he died she could not bring herself to cook complicated meals for herself, and lived on foods she found comforting and convenient – which was usually jacket potatoes – without thinking of what this was doing to her diet.

Now she has been introduced to the 200 foods and has realised her dependence on potatoes, she thinks more about what to cook, instead of just eating anything to hand. She now feels well, has more self-confidence, and does not have those aches and pains any more. She has much more energy and says that she is fast becoming a 'health nut'!

The Food Addict's Diet is just what we need to make being a woman a less distressing experience. If every woman made sure that she ate well, then she could avoid a great many female ailments.

CHAPTER 13
Put an End to Bingeing

This chapter assumes that you are following the four zero plan, even if you find it hard to follow for long without bingeing on food. I hope that you have found that you binge less often now that your strongest food addictions are kept under control by the Food Addict's Diet. With the help of the advice in this chapter you can now make long-term diet and lifestyle changes to stop bingeing completely, and find out how to break binges if they still occur from time to time.

BINGE AND OVERDOSE

Binges are overdoses of food, and we have mentioned them already in other chapters. The zero plan will have already pinpointed the four foods most people take as overdoses; food-drug combinations commonly overdosed were discussed in Chapter 10 (see pages 161–71); and any other addictions created by food intolerance were covered in Chapter 11 (pages 181–4). In Chapter 12 there was an explanation of why some women notice changes in appetite during their monthly cycle (see pages 189–90). If you have a tendency to binge, even occasionally, all this advice should have already helped to reduce the number of times it happens.

COMPULSIVE EATING

In this chapter I shall call the phenomenon of bingeing 'compulsive eating'. The element of compulsion is important here; this is the need to cram food into your mouth when you know you do not need it, but feel that you simply *must* have it. This is how most people feel during a binge.

The Food Addict's Diet helps people to control their appetite whether their cravings are almost imperceptible or whether they have come to rule their appetite completely. Binges occur when eating gets out of control and addictive cravings for certain foods overwhelm your natural hungers (pages 91–2).

ARE YOU A COMPULSIVE EATER?

Take a look at the following statements. If any of these apply to you, either occasionally or every day of your life, answer 'yes'.

1. I crave for food.
2. I am afraid when my appetite is out of my control
3. I have great difficulty keeping my eating habits under my control.
4. I have a constant feeling of hunger that food does not satisfy.
5. When I start eating I am unable to stop.

If you have answered 'yes' to any of these, you are not a freak of nature, depraved or crazy: you are just a food addict.

COPING WITH THE PROBLEMS OF COMPULSIVE EATING

The principal problem with compulsive eating is the danger of putting on weight, and there are three ways in which compulsive eaters tend to deal with this.

A rapid weight gain because of overeating is often

shortly followed by a drastic slimming diet to undo the damage. This is sometimes called the 'binge/fast cycle', and was a common problem among the trials candidates.

Less commonly, the binger takes steps to get rid of the food almost immediately, including vomiting and taking laxatives: this is known as bulimia. Four of the 100 trials applicants were bulimics, including Pamela, whom you met on page 11. (We will deal in more detail with the vomiting later, on page 208.)

More rarely still, the binger manages to bring her cravings for food under control by fasting, but then becomes frightened to reawaken them and stops eating: this is anorexia nervosa, and it seems also to have its roots in compulsive eating and food addiction. Although no one suffering with anorexia applied to join the trials, three of my candidates told me that they had endured episodes of anorexia in the past, and described their feelings to me in detail. All three of them individually described how they became obsessive about food in a desperate effort to keep control, and eventually refused to eat anything for some time. One candidate was reduced to five stones in weight and spent four months in hospital. In each case, their past lives showed various signs of addiction: one was a recovered drug addict, another had once been an alcoholic, and when I met them they were all very strongly addicted to the four zero foods.

Christine: A typical compulsive eater

Let's meet Christine, who could not understand her own eating behaviour, and did not realise that her problem was compulsive eating.

The wife of a jobbing builder, Christine lives on the edge of a large town in an unfriendly suburb. Her son, now aged twenty, has left home to live with his girlfriend, leaving Christine at home on her own, with little to do.

Christine is about forty pounds overweight, and has

tried various diets in the past, but she rarely manages to follow any diet for longer than a few days. She is a typical compulsive eater, planning binges in advance, eating guiltily and in secret.

She often makes chocolate cake, knowing all the time that she will not be able to resist it and will eat it all on her own. She will not answer the door while she is eating, but will rush upstairs to the bathroom, and hide there until the visitors go away. If her husband answers the door she then emerges normally and comes down to speak to them. After they have gone she will go into the kitchen and secretly begin to eat the cake again, hiding it if her husband comes near, until it is all gone.

Later on we will see how Christine began to understand her eating behaviour and put an end to her secret binges on cake mainly because of her change of attitude to food addiction.

THE IMPORTANCE OF YOUR ATTITUDE

There are two important elements to any binge – the foods you eat and the way you feel about the food you have eaten. Far too many people think compulsive eating is merely an obsession with body weight. This is true, but the obsession is created by a ravenous hunger that will not be quieted. There is no need to blame yourself for this problem: it arose not from a lack of will power but from your addictive cravings for food.

GUILTY EATING

Compulsive eating can range from a tendency to snatch secret guilty snacks between meals to an overwhelming craving that no amount of food can satisfy. The scale of the problem depends not upon the amount of food taken, but upon the amount of guilt that goes with it.

How you feel about a binge can range from a slight feeling of guilt to almost total despair, and this depends

200

on how long you have had the problem and how extreme your cravings are.

A NEGATIVE VIEW OF FOOD

Most compulsive eaters seem eventually to develop a negative view of their food. A lifetime of the binge/fast cycle makes eating any kind of food into a threat to their slimming efforts. The ex-anorexics I spoke to (see page 199) had at the time of their anorexia seen all food as a terrible threat to their figure, even though they were already quite thin. It is common knowledge that many anorexics have a career where slimness and lightness is essential, such as dancing and photographic modelling, and eat very little in perpetual fear of gaining weight.

A LIVING NIGHTMARE

The constant craving for food can trigger off binges that are alarming in their ferocity and shamelessness, even driving the poor binger into the kitchen rubbish bin for scraps like a starving vagrant. The desperate desire to be slim and in control sends almost every binger off on a desperate search for cure at any cost. After the initial joyful moments of success, every new slimming diet breaks down, bringing yet another demoralising experience of failure.

A great many compulsive eaters have some deep-rooted psychological problem, stemming from traumatic experiences in the past, such as rape, abortion, sexual abuse or enforced starvation, and all too often during psychotherapy they are forced to face up to deep-seated personal problems while feeling weak, ill and panicky as a result of their eating disorder. One of the compulsive eaters I met during the trials described the past sixteen years of bulimia as 'a living nightmare'.

Christine learns to laugh

Christine, our cake-eating compulsive eater, tried the four zero plan many times before she got it right. The first time she stuck with it for five days was a complete revelation to her, as she found that she was strongly addicted to wheat-based foods, and she told me that the feeling she had when she gave up wheat was just like giving up smoking cigarettes.

Christine's first attempt at the zero plan lasted less than a week, but before she could lapse into despair I introduced her to the restart plan. She made a new beginning the next Monday but lapsed again on the Friday. This became a weekly pattern until I discovered that she baked cakes ready for the weekend every Friday and could never resist them for long: she was deliberately testing her resolve and losing!

The next week she survived a weekend by not baking any cakes and eating rye bread and honey instead of cake, but early the next week she yielded to a Danish pastry at a cafe.

Finally, after many attempts at the four zero plan, a remarkable thing happened: she began to laugh at herself and her addiction to cakes and pastries – something that was quite out of character, for she was normally a serious person. I took this as a sign that at last she was coming to terms with her addiction to wheat, and it was.

From then on she became much more attentive to her diet, more careful of avoiding the four zeros, and managed to stay for weeks at a time on the Food Addict's Diet, giving in to cakes and pastries only occasionally at tea parties. She has now lost ten pounds without really trying and, as far as I know, her secret, guilty cake-eating sessions are over for good.

This case study illustrates very well how important a change of attitude is in beating compulsive eating, but there are also many other practical steps you can take to end your binges for ever.

PUT AN END TO BINGEING

Avoid the four zeros

Think of your last binge and make a list of the foods you ate in the spaces below and put a ring around any zero foods contained in them:

Binge food	*Zero foods present*
....	wheat/sugar/potato/milk
....	wheat/sugar/potato/milk
....	wheat/sugar/potato/milk
....	wheat/sugar/potato/milk
....	wheat/sugar/potato/milk
....	wheat/sugar/potato/milk
....	wheat/sugar/potato/milk

If you still feel a yen for the four zeros from time to time, concentrate on completely avoiding the four zeros as your first step.

Binges start in the shops, so never buy foods you know you can't resist just to test your resolve: you know your resolve will not be able to take it! From now on let no excuse allow you to take even a tiny fragment of the four zero foods, and concentrate on the rest of the 200 foods to build your menus.

Remove all traces of the zeros from the house, and if necessary put the whole family on to the zero plan (see pages 212–20). Tell your friends you are not allowed to touch the four zeros, and use food intolerance as an excuse if it helps. Avoid restaurants where the four zeros are served and tell yourself they are DANGER!

YOUR NEW BINGE FOODS

If none of your binge foods now contain the four zero foods, you have made an important first step towards an end to bingeing for good. Take a good look at the type of food you now choose to binge upon. Whatever it is, it is likely to be easy to swallow, sweet-tasting and concentrated, because this kind of food is easiest to eat in large quantities.

You chose your binge food with great care: it must be ready to eat and is rarely cooked first, unless it can be cooked quickly, like custard. Custards and other sloppy foods are easy to swallow and slip down easily, and fresh and dried fruits are favourites because they provide the sweet taste that keeps you wanting more and more.

Crisp fresh fruit and raw vegetables are tiring to chew after a while, so use these as binge food now. Watery, fibre-rich foods such as thick vegetable soups or stewed dried fruit are very filling, so use these as your new binge food and see how soon you are full, almost to bursting point.

EAT WELL

Don't go without food for too long, for an empty stomach is your enemy: have a good breakfast and a good lunch. Keep busy at night and allow yourself a healthy snack or a small meal every two hours of the day at first, gradually cutting down your food in the evening first and working back through the day.

CHANGE YOUR EATING BEHAVIOUR

Just as the smuggler must declare his goods, so you must now declare your food, so publicise what you are eating by putting it on a plate and making an 'occasion' out of eating it. Do not nibble in secret: prepare a plateful of good food and take it into the family room to eat in full view of everyone else. If you live alone, you can try to look into a mirror as you eat, or invite someone in to eat with you as often as you can.

CHEW ON YOUR MISTAKES

If you do happen to be tempted to eat a food you know triggers off a binge, do not spit the food out, but accept it, telling yourself that it is food to nourish you and give you energy, and need not be a guilty secret. Keep it and chew it – not two chews and down the throat, *really* chew it! Good chewing should mash food to a pulp and mix it well with saliva. It should be so well mixed that you can hardly stop yourself swallowing it. If you are tense, tired, very hungry, or even panicking it is hard to remember to chew, but do try.

KEEP UP THE THERAPY

Following the plan combines well with counselling sessions of some kind: at home you can begin to bring your cravings under your control, and during the counselling sessions you can begin to come to terms with your past. Use every kind of help you can obtain to support you and keep you going.

KEEP CRAVINGS IN PERSPECTIVE

You may still crave food, but your cravings for food are not constant every day. They come and go, and there are some foods that you crave and others that you do not. Gradually, as you continue on the Food Addict's Diet, you will find that you have a few days here and there when your cravings are almost non-existent!

LOSING WEIGHT

Gradually you will feel your health improving. All kinds of nervous symptoms and other physical effects will have diminished with the help of your new healthy diet, and now you will be able to think more sensibly about your weight. It may be better to allow your weight to drop naturally as your food intake stabilises, so do not try to slim too soon.

The Food Addict's Diet will act as a healthy maintenance diet and will keep your weight steady until you feel you can cope with a slimming diet. When you start slimming do not count calories, or you will run the risk of getting obsessed again with your food allowances. Use one of the other slimming options, especially the grain-free option or the 'slim week' (pages 144–8).

BE A WINNER

Winners' Groups (see page 301) are a good place for compulsive eaters to find comfort and reassurance. Here you can meet with others who are fighting the weight-loss battle and see how your problem, far from being an intractable psychological disorder, is simply a very extreme example of a problem experienced by so many tens of thousands of people: controlling the appetite.

IF YOU STILL BINGE

If you still binge from time to time, don't worry. Like any other addiction, it will tend to beckon you back in times of stress. Every time you give in to your cravings, remember that this happens often enough to every food addict, and you are no worse than anyone else. Use the restart plan to get back in control. Gradually, as you give in and restart, time and time again, you will find yourself losing the fear of losing control which is so much part of your problem.

PRACTICAL TIPS

Use your balance hunger
During a binge remember to use your balance hunger, and choose one single basic ingredient to eat. Do not vary the ingredients during the binge, so that your balance hunger will act as a natural 'switch-off'. Try using raisins, dates or figs, until you feel genuinely nauseated by the amount you have eaten, and use that feeling to help you to stop eating.

How to stop that binge

Now the binge has started, you are in a kind of coma: you are hardly aware of what is going on around you. You are completely lost in satisfying that overwhelming need to stuff food into your mouth. Just for a fraction of a second, let reality creep back. THINK.

Now become aware of the food in your mouth. It is, after all, only food, rich in nutrients for you and your body. Keep it in your mouth as long as you can, and work on it. Taste how delicious it is. Savour it and feel saliva flowing. Begin to chew it *properly*. Try to keep it in your mouth as long as you can. Roll the food around the mouth until it is moist with all the large pieces broken down; you will by now be desperate to swallow it!

After swallowing, clean your mouth as carefully as you can using your tongue. This will send some extra saliva down to help the last mouthful. By helping the saliva to flow you are encouraging your digestion to behave normally. Let it cover your food completely, and let a fair amount of it get swallowed with the food. An acid fruit drink taken during a binge, and held in the mouth for as long as you can, will stimulate a lot of saliva and kill the taste of the binge food.

While you are doing this, move away from the food area, carrying some more of the *same* food with you. If you can, put your coat on and go outside into the street and walk, still carrying the food. Once you have walked a little way, you can eat it. If there are people around, try even then to eat it publicly, even if you feel a fool.

Just take a little bite and chew it as carefully as you can and keep it in your mouth for as long as you possibly can. By now the effect of consciously thinking of your food, the saliva coating it and the volume of food in your stomach will have begun to switch off your hunger. Walk until the craving feeling begins to die down, which could take about half an hour. (If you cannot leave the house, you can achieve almost the same effect by going into another room instead of outside.)

I know that binges take place in a dream world where

reality is far away but just being aware of your mouth will drag you into the present moment and remind you to chew: remember, practice makes perfect. This method has already been found useful for several candidates during the trials, one of whom met her neighbour in the street after a binge on cold sausages, and ended up feeding the sausages she was carrying to the neighbour's dog, which could be an interesting new way to put an end to a binge!

ARE YOU ADDICTED TO BINGEING ITSELF?

Hooked on vomiting

If you vomit after a binge to rid yourself of the food you have eaten, then you have found a way to binge without getting fat. If you have been vomiting frequently, no doubt your teeth are beginning to rot from the stomach acids in your mouth. If you find you cannot tolerate any large meal without wanting to vomit it out of the way, then you have a problem.

Not only is there the true hunger you feel because your stomach is empty again, but your digestion is probably in such a mess by now that you are probably getting very little nourishment from the food you do keep down. This is probably triggering off deficiency cravings to add to your addictive cravings and creating an enormous and overwhelming desire to eat (see page 91).

The vomiting used to solve a problem, but it is now a problem in itself. Think hard about the relief and satisfaction bingeing and vomiting gives you and realise that you binge deliberately, just so that you can be sick at the end of it. Then you can disgorge many frustrations and angers along with the vomited binge food, leaving you empty and drained. Just like any other addict after a fix, you are somehow now able to cope with life again – until the next fix.

Like so many other forms of self-abuse, episodes of bulimia can bring feelings of relief and satisfaction.

The overload of food in your stomach and the forced vomiting afterwards creates an enormous amount of stress, which releases our old friends the endorphins, and this is how you can become hooked on the whole idea, and find it hard to stop (see pages 81–2).

If you decide to put a stop to the vomiting after a binge you must expect a slight weight gain as the first effect, but do not panic: you have the rest of your life to lose weight again with the help of the four zero plan plus the slimming options on pages 144–58.

If you have been vomiting frequently you may find it unbearable to feel at all full, as this triggers off an impulse to be sick and a feeling of panic. The way round this is to avoid large meals and take small snacks many times a day, making them nourishing and varied with plenty of raw food. Then gradually increase the size of your meals until you can tolerate a main meal.

Remember that if you have planned your binge with vomiting in mind you are probably addicted to that sense of relief and satisfaction. Read again the stages of overcoming an addiction (pages 87–9). Expect to feel deprived after a while, and to feel the urge to binge again when you are under stress. Recognise these feelings when they occur and this will help enormously, then try to find another, safer method of coping with the stresses in your life.

Abuse of laxatives

Compulsive eaters often use laxatives to get rid of their food as fast as possible, sometimes combined with vomiting.

Unfortunately, long-term abuse of laxatives can upset the natural balance of bacteria in your gut, which can lead to all kinds of other digestive problems, including a noisily rumbling stomach or excessive flatulence. Also, taking laxatives constantly over a long period can create a distended abdomen: this protrudes and is hard to pull in, and increases the effects of any weight gain still further. Abuse of laxatives can also create nutritional deficiencies, for the goodness in your food is not absorbed properly owing to disturbances in your digestion.

If you decide to stop taking laxatives remember that your nutritional deficiencies will remain until you begin to build up your health by eating as much variety as you can of fresh, real whole food. You can help the situation with some food supplements, particularly the minerals and B vitamins. You must also expect a short period of readjustment while your digestive system returns to normal, and this may take the form of constipation: if so, do not take more laxatives, but eat as much high-fibre food as you can in the form of fresh fruits and vegetables, which will be easier for your digestive system to cope with than cereal bran.

A LINK BETWEEN COMPULSIVE EATING AND FOOD INTOLERANCE

The symptoms that often accompany eating disorders of various kinds, such as anxiety, headaches, a racing pulse, and various digestive disorders, are usually put down to malnutrition. However, they are also symptoms of food intolerance (see the list on pages 41–3) and will respond to the some of the treatments available for allergies and food intolerance. (As we have already established the link between addictive cravings and food intolerance, I do not find this at all surprising.) If you happen to have access to a reputable allergy therapist specialising in treating food intolerance, you may find some of his methods helpful as an additional benefit.

I know of at least one bulimic who has been very successfully treated by methods usually reserved for those suffering from food intolerance. Dr Jean Munroe of Abbots Langley hospital told me during an interesting discussion with her that one patient with a long history of bulimia was successfully treated by being given a range of desensitising drops for about twenty everyday foods. These drops are used at Dr Munroe's clinic to combat the symptoms of food intolerance, but in this case the drops had the effect of killing this woman's cravings for these foods. As a result, she was able to eat a balanced diet based on these twenty ingredients, and made a good recovery.

The four zero experiment has already proved to you that there is a simple, physical reason why you crave food, and the four zero plan is a practical way to overcome your cravings. As you isolate your own addictions and bring them under control, the number of times you binge will slowly diminish until you have no further need to binge at all. This may be a long hard road for you, but the Food Addict's Diet will help you, every step of the way.

CHAPTER 14
Feeding the Family

This chapter will show you how the three-week experiment can be a useful way to see to what extent other members of your family are addicted to, or intolerant of, their food. The tendency to food intolerance is an inherited trait, and if you or your partner show signs of it, then your children are probably also reacting in some way to their food.

Throughout this chapter I have assumed that you have tried the four zero experiment yourself; if you have not, then please do so before introducing the diet to anyone else, even if you do not suffer from excess weight or any of the health problems listed on pages 41–3. You will be better able to introduce this new way of eating to others if you have experienced it for yourself, and have become familiar with the changes that are required in shopping and cooking.

This chapter will provide you with some special advice for when you try the experiment with your partner or children. Even if you found the experiment a very useful and revealing experience yourself, it is less easy to involve others in trying it out, even if they are badly in need of a change of diet. Their addictions will make them very sceptical and resistant to the idea of giving up the four zero foods, and much of the advice given here is designed to help you to understand and overcome this resistance.

YOUR CHILD'S FOOD ADDICTIONS

NOTE: Throughout this section I have referred to a male child and a female parent. This is purely for convenience and does not imply that daughters have no problems or that fathers never prepare food for their children.

This section will deal with three specific diet-related problems in children: first, overeating and being overweight; secondly, allergic reactions and intolerance to food; and lastly, behaviour problems and hyperactivity – both of which are now widely accepted as being closely related to food intolerance and other chemical allergies.

These problems can be helped greatly by a change of diet, but this is not easy, partly because of social pressures. Having tried the experiment yourself, you will already know how such pressures can affect your eating habits, and they are every bit as strong upon your child. Owing to his immature personality he is extremely vulnerable to them, and they may be the principal reason why he has become a food addict. A great deal of effort on your part will have to be spent upon dealing with these outside pressures and relieving them where you can, so that you can begin to change your child's diet.

There are many pressures moulding the way children eat, but here we will focus on three of the strongest: you as his parent telling him what to eat, his friends as his peer group persuading him to conform with them, and television food advertisements – which play on a child's love of sweet tastes, exciting textures, colour and excitement.

TEACHING CHILDREN HOW TO EAT

Parents are the principal influence on any child's diet: they select the range of food to be offered, choose the recipe to prepare it, present it to the child, and cajole him into eating it when he is unwilling to try. To this extent, food addictions are 'inherited', for mothers tend to feed their children only the foods they enjoy, and are less likely to serve dishes that they dislike. In this way, food tastes are handed down through families, often for several generations.

Parental pressure can be turned to good effect, though, for parents can turn the family home into a training ground for healthy eating. By giving your child a healthy, varied diet such as the Food Addict's Diet with all kinds of unusual foods being served, prejudices against certain foods – such as 'greens' – will soon be overcome.

The myth of 'children's food'

There is no 'children's food': there is just food. Children are capable of eating just the same foods as adults (with the possible exception of highly spiced dishes and hard foods such as nuts, which a young child may be unable to chew properly).

Some parents have been led to believe that their offspring need a different kind of diet from adults, with plenty of high-calorie food such as crisps or sweets to provide them with energy. Children grow very fast, and certainly do need enough calories, but they should be given lots of fresh, real, varied, whole food to provide for all their nutritional needs.

If your child is listless and lacking in energy he may be deficient in some vital nutrients such as iron or B vitamins, or even intolerant to the foods you give him every day. If that is so, he will continue to lack energy as long as you give him the same repetitive round of his favourite foods. The changes you made in your own diet when you began the Food Addict's Diet brought you a new burst of energy, and it will do the same for your child.

Softly, softly!

Children often reject foods that are unfamiliar, but that should not make it impossible to feed them a healthy, varied diet. Children are very suspicious of new foods, and so any changes in a child's diet must be made slowly and almost imperceptibly until the new flavour has been accepted. Take, for example, the recipe on page 265 for Shepherd's Parsnip Pie: this has a topping made from puréed parsnip instead of potato. If you were suddenly to offer parsnip topping to your child, who was expecting to taste the familiar flavour of potato, he would naturally reject it. However, if you slowly mix a little more parsnip into the potato topping every time you make this dish, he will gradually become familiar with the flavour and will begin to enjoy its sweet taste.

You can make a child fussy about his food by constantly serving him the same small group of 'children's recipes', and eventually any slightly unfamiliar flavour will be rejected at once. This could be how you became a food addict long ago, and how your child in turn will eventually begin to crave his favourites. In fact, he is probably already well on the way to becoming addicted to the four zeros, for every day of his life so far he is almost certain to have eaten wheat, potatoes, milk and sugar in some form or other.

Beat hunger with an extra meal

Be aware of the role of hunger in your child's need for snacks and treats. To put a stop to those daily trips to the sweet shop after school, consider introducing an extra meal into the day. School-age children are growing fast and are often genuinely hungry, particularly just after school, and it is better to satisfy that hunger with good food rather than snacks. So, when he comes home from school, have a nourishing snack ready for him to eat at once, and serve his main meal a little later in the evening. In this way you can bridge that hungry gap before tea without using sweets and biscuits.

Give them good food as snacks

Children love to snack, and you can use snacks as a way of introducing new textures and tastes. As soon as your

215

child is able to chew them properly, introduce him to a variety of raw fruits and vegetables and use them often as a snack, cut into strips or interesting shapes. Dried fruits, nuts for the older children, and seeds can be bought in packets in place of sweets. Rye crispbreads and oatcakes, and non-wheat home-made biscuits such as flapjacks (see recipes, page 283) are just as tasty and pleasant to eat as crisps or biscuits, and much cheaper!

COPING WITH PEER PRESSURE

Peer pressure – that is, the desire to do just the same as his friends – is a major force in your child's upbringing. He tends to imitate his contemporaries and others whom he admires. If he changes his diet in any way your child will have to deal with the sneers of his friends in exactly the same way as you had to risk being labelled a 'health freak' when you began the four zero experiment. If you can make the changes in your child's diet subtle and slow, he and his friends will hardly notice. When they come to tea, make them a tasty, interesting meal of some of the less usual foods and see how much they enjoy them!

If your child is aged between nine and fourteen, where peer-group pressure is at its strongest and self-confidence at its weakest, provide your child with an interesting and varied selection of healthy foods in his lunch box every day. (Recipe suggestions can be found on pages 257–8.) He may even set a new trend among his friends, and thus turn peer pressure to good effect!

ADDICTIONS AND ADVERTISING

While we worry about sex and violence on television, are we really paying enough attention to the effects of food advertising on our children's eating habits? Food advertisements carry all kinds of implicit messages about the fun of confectionery, the taste and texture of crisps, and the excitement of breakfast cereals, and this is powerful stuff.

Food companies are in the business of increasing sales rather than health education, and they tend to feed and maintain our addictions by emphasising the happiness and satisfactions to be gained from their products. Advertising companies know our addictions and play them for all they are worth. My own family found that over three evenings about 85 per cent of food products advertised between 4 p.m. and 9 p.m. were made with at least one of the four zero foods. The remaining 15 per cent were mainly alcoholic drinks, margarine and fruit juices.

TRYING THE EXPERIMENT WITH YOUR CHILD

PROBLEMS GETTING STARTED

If he resists very strongly the whole idea of the zero plan and becomes unhappy or defiant, then forget the diet for a while and carry on with the gradual changes you are making to a more varied diet. As the dependence on his favourites begins to diminish, then so too will his addictions and, in turn, his resistance to trying the experiment.

BE PREPARED

Don't rush it! I suggest that you spend at least three weeks preparing your child for the change of diet. The more small changes you can introduce now the easier the experiment will be for everyone. You have more to do this time than shop for interesting alternative foods: you also have to ease your child into a new way of eating and lay the foundations for his new diet.

Help him to become aware of what he eats

Make a food diary for your child, using a similar form to the one shown on pages 75–6. This will show you how limited his diet is, and the foods he is hooked on. Teach him to read the labels on packaged foods: we know already from the trials that children find this fun, and they are often curious about the long chemical names of food additives when they try to pronounce them! They can also learn to score their own diet and increase their score, perhaps in competition with other members of the family. (One grandmother I know who attempted to compete with her granddaughter in this way learned a salutary lesson about how narrow her own diet had become!)

Introduce the other sources of calcium

Try the other animal milks for a change, and reduce your child's dependence on milk by changing the foods you serve at breakfast (see recipes, pages 251-5) and having cold drinks in place of tea or coffee. It is not a good idea to give your child caffeine drinks in any case, as they can lead to an addiction and cause further problems (see pages 168-71). Begin to feed your child non-dairy high-calcium foods daily until he is familiar with them (see the Calci-Counter on pages 286-94).

Young children on the plan

If a very young child shows symptoms of allergy or food intolerance, be careful if you try the plan on them to alleviate their symptoms. Removing wheat, sugar and potatoes from a young child's diet should cause no nutritional problem providing they are replaced with plenty of other high-energy foods that are not too high in fibre. However, young children, especially those under five, are very dependent upon cows' milk for calcium, and will need a calcium supplement if you find that they also react to sheep's or goats' milk. In that case I would advise you to take this book to your doctor, tell him what you intend to do and why, and ask him to prescribe a suitable calcium supplement.

Unfortunately, the training of doctors more or less ignores nutrition so it is not appropriate to ask your doctor how to feed your child. Instead, ask for an appointment with a dietitian, who will be able to advise you about which of the other animal and seed milks are safe to use for young children. Do not give a young child soya milk from the health-food shop as his only calcium source: soya milk is a good healthy protein drink, but it is not a good source of calcium.

The day before you start
Make out an assessment form similar to the form on pages 112–16 and fill it in carefully, recording all the details you can about your child's particular problem. Make sure that there is a plentiful supply of alternative foods for your child, especially in the first few days of the experiment.

The three weeks on the plan
Follow the instructions as given on pages 117–31 and make sure that your child has plenty of interesting alternative foods to eat in the first week. Take it gently, and start by offering substitutes for the four zeros and extra fruit as a treat, which most children enjoy. If he doesn't like the new milk, then don't bother with cereals at all, or limit them to once a week.

The attitude of others
Regardless of why your child is trying this diet, tell him, his teacher and those around him that he is on a special diet to test for food intolerance, which hopefully will produce an attitude of support and sympathy from other adults, rather than impatient derision – which I have seen all too often aimed at children when they refuse to eat what is on their plate.

Keep it polite
If you are still avoiding the four zero foods because of your own addictions, you probably cope with eating out by politely accepting the food that is offered and dealing with its effects on your cravings later: now your child will have to learn to do the same.

You must be careful not to have him labelled as 'difficult' by irritated mothers, confronted by a child who says he is 'not allowed' to eat anything on the table. Help him to see how his cravings can be activated by an overdose of his favourites, but remind him often that when he eats out a small lapse is quite OK.

Be relaxed about his lapses

He will probably give in again and again until the day he manages to stick with the plan, and even then he will never be absolutely consistent, any more than you were when you first tried it; so do not drive him into secret eating by being angry or dictatorial: remember that you too were once a victim to your addictive cravings.

In my experience, some children can take the four zero experiment very seriously indeed, and become quite worried about the effects of eating even a little of their banned foods. This makes life unnecessarily difficult for everyone, so cultivate a relaxed attitude to lapsing from the plan at all times. This diet can produce many good effects, but if it just makes your child over-anxious about his food the good effects will soon be cancelled out.

OVERWEIGHT CHILDREN

The basic four zero plan is a good maintenance diet for children who are overweight, and they can use it for an extended period while they grow out of their weight problem. I suggest that as a first step you try the plan for three weeks and then assess progress.

NOTE: Do not try the rest test (pages 135–6), because your child may not be able to cope with the sudden surge in his addictive cravings. There are bound to be lapses in any case that will demonstrate his addictive cravings quite clearly enough. Older children who lose sight of the point of the diet after a while can try the rest test to see for themselves how much progress they have made in controlling their food consumption. The restart plan (pages 136–8) can be useful if things break down entirely to get everyone going again.

THE DAY BEFORE YOU START

Weigh and measure your child carefully, and note the results on the measurement chart below. This form can be copied by hand or photocopied for use with other children in your family.

MEASUREMENT CHART

Child's name ....
Dates: Start of experiment: ..../..../19....
       End of experiment: ..../..../19....

Measurements	Changes after three weeks (+ or −)
Height ....ft....in (....cm)	....in/cm
Weight ....st....lb (....kg)	....lb/kg
Body measurements:	
Chest ....in/....cm	....in/cm
Waist ....in/....cm	....in/cm
Hips ....in/....cm	....in/cm
Thighs	
right ....in/....cm	....in/cm
left ....in/....cm	....in/cm
Upper arms	
right ....in/....cm	....in/m
left ....in/....cm	....in/cm

THREE WEEKS ON THE PLAN

Do not tell everyone that your child is 'slimming', because this may embarrass him: say that he is being tested for food intolerance (see page 219).

Never let your child feel deprived, and he will stay happy on the diet. He can eat as much as he likes of the foods that are not banned, so he can take a lunch box to school stuffed with a good filling meal made from allowed ingredients (see packed lunch suggestions on pages 257–8).

DURING THE THIRD WEEK

Make a food diary using a form similar to the one on pages 75–6 and use it to assess how varied your child's diet now is, how many times he lapses, and which foods attract him particularly. Discuss the results with him if he is old enough.

Measure him again and see how he is doing at the end of the third week. Mark the results on the chart on page 221 with a plus (+) for a gain and a minus (−) for a loss.

ASSESSING RESULTS

Keep reminding your child that to be successful on this diet he will not need to lose weight, but he must reduce his food consumption enough not to gain weight. Therefore if his weight remains constant that can be a cause for celebration and reward. As time passes he will lose body fat even if he loses no weight at all, so pay particular attention to those small changes in his body measurements. They will be at their greatest if he is growing very fast, and children do not grow evenly, so the changes will vary enormously from week to week.

WHERE NEXT?

Your own experiences on the experiment and after will have shown you how the zero plan enables you to eat well without gaining weight. Now you have a clearer idea of which foods your child cannot control, work hard to keep them out of this life, and let any zero foods he can keep under control creep back into his diet in small doses – but do not allow them to take over from all the other new foods you have introduced.

I do not recommend that you use the slimming options on pages 144–58 with your child while he is still growing. He does not need to take any further steps to slim down: let nature take care of that while you feed him a varied and satisfying diet of real, whole foods.

To show you the many ways in which the plan can help an overweight child, meet Peter.

Peter slims down with the four zero plan

When I met Peter he was twelve years old, five foot six inches tall, and two stones above the correct weight for his height. He agreed to try the four zero plan for three weeks because it was put to him simply as a short-term experiment.

He started the diet with characteristic enthusiasm, and soon developed a liking for dates and dried apricots, which he ate copiously at first. His parents were worried about his calcium intake, so he was given a supplement to take daily. During the first week he suffered bouts of diarrhoea and flatulence, and he felt very tired. This was probably withdrawal, but his parents became a little worried. Even so he had a good appetite, and was eating freely of the allowed foods, so we carried on. Gradually his energy increased, and by the end of the second week he was feeling very well and had lost four pounds in weight and an inch off his waist and hips. He was amazed, because he had been eating so much.

On the Monday of the third week he felt bored with the diet and missed his usual sweets. That evening he bought some, and the moment he ate one he wanted the entire packet. This surprised him, because he thought he could now control his consumption of sugar, but now his sugar addiction was made clear to him, and obviously he would have to avoid sugar entirely while he was trying to keep his food consumption down.

He had always suffered from constipation, but by the end of three weeks on the plan this was no longer a problem. He had more energy and felt calmer, although he had never been a nervous child. His demeanour was now more confident, and even his teachers noticed it.

Nine months later on his thirteenth birthday he had lost seven pounds since the start of the experiment, had grown two inches in height, and had lost a total of three inches off his waist, two inches off his thighs and an inch from his upper arms, where the fat is fast being replaced by muscle. He was no longer regarded as a 'fatty', but considered by everyone as 'well-built', like his father, which pleased him immensely. He even took a narrower shoe fitting, which made it easier to buy him footwear.

When I spoke to him recently Peter had so far managed to avoid sugar almost totally, but he was still very easily tempted by cheese and other dairy products. He makes stir-fries and soup for himself after school and he wants to be a chef when he eventually leaves. Not only that, but as a result of repeated requests from his parents, soup, pâtés, rye crispbreads and boiled rice now appear on the menu at his school from time to time.

CHILDREN WITH FOOD INTOLERANCE AND OTHER ALLERGIES

As we discovered on page 175, the tendency to react to all kinds of other substances in the environment can be inherited. There are some families that are 'atopic', and where reactions to all kinds of things, including stress, are manifested in various ways: as allergies, such as eczema or asthma, or as food intolerance, which can produce any of the symptoms listed on pages 41–3. Therefore, if you found that you were intolerant to your food when you tried the experiment, look closely at your child's health and see if he displays any symptoms. If he does, see if three weeks on the zero plan brings about an improvement.

This section will deal with two problems that are specifically related to children: allergies such as asthma, eczema, hives, and hay fever, and the effects of food intolerance on concentration and behaviour.

REDUCING THE LOAD

You can reduce the total load on your child and the occurrence of his symptoms in several ways even before you begin to change his diet (see pages 175–7). Vary his diet as much as you can, so that no single food is repeated too often. Build up his health with plenty of good healthy foods, a daily multivitamin and mineral supplement, rest, fresh air and regular gentle exercise. Aim at all times to give your child real, natural whole food as free from additives as possible, and eliminate as many chemicals from his environment as you can (see pages 180–1). Reduce any stress on him by clearing up any trouble at school and reassuring him about his fears and failings.

TRYING THE PLAN

Put your child on the plan for three weeks at first, as we did for excess weight (see pages 220–22), and then assess the results. If the change of diet seems to be helping, carry on with it, but notice when there are lapses if his symptoms get worse, and which foods are most likely to be the cause of the trouble. There are more details below that are specific to each problem.

ALLERGIES

Chronic symptoms

Eczema is a common chronic symptom in children, and is often aggravated by food intolerance. So add eggs, oranges and tomatoes to your list of zero foods, for they are common culprits in children's allergies, and they form an integral part of the dishes we serve as 'children's food' (see page 214). This step can also be taken if your child shows any of the food intolerance symptoms listed on pages 41-3.

When your child's symptoms begin to calm down, breaking the diet will probably trigger them off again. Each time this happens your child is learning an important lesson. Chronic reactions tend to continue for many years, and so this lesson needs to be learned early, for there will always be a tendency to become addicted to the food or substance that causes the reaction.

Acute reactions
If you practise the plan occasionally with your child at times when his symptoms have faded away, then you will both know just what to do when 'reaction time' comes round again, such as the hay fever season.

Hay fever and exams
If you have a teenager with hay fever who is sitting exams, begin the diet well before exam week to get through withdrawal and deprivation before exams begin. Make sure that your child understands the importance of staying with the diet rigidly while sitting his exams. There are various homoeopathic remedies that do not cause drowsiness and will calm hay fever reactions, and a large dose of Vitamin C (1 g) will keep the lid on things when the pollen count is very high, especially in the late evening when reactions are often at their worst.

Reduce the reaction
Even if the diet gives little result, always beware of overdoses, for they can help to precipitate reactions by increasing stress. Take any steps you can to reduce the load on your child (see page 225). In any case, Vitamin C is a way to help calm an acute allergic reaction. You cannot overdose on this vitamin, but do not give your child more than 2 g in twenty-four hours as it can cause diarrhoea if given in large quantities.

TANTRUMS

Tantrums in children can arise directly out of addictive cravings, as we discovered during the trials.

Stephanie

Stephanie, a seven-year-old who drank nothing but cola drinks, threw a tantrum at least once a day, often at mealtimes. Her mother thought that this might be a kind of hyperactivity and decided to try the experiment. She bought sugar-free, caffeine-free cola drinks for Stephanie when the experiment began and offered her other fruit drinks as well to increase the variety in her diet. Stephanie became less and less angry about everything, including being denied her cola drink, and her mother realised then that Stephanie had been hooked on caffeine, and the tantrums were an expression of her addictive cravings.

She bought some fizzy sugar-free apple juice and presented it to Stephanie with much ceremony as a 'special treat'. Stephanie now looks upon this as her 'own special drink' and at first would have no other. Since she began avoiding her cola drinks Stephanie has never thrown another tantrum of any kind. To prevent any further tantrums should this new favourite drink not be available, we experimented with other fruit juices mixed with fizzy mineral water, and Stephanie soon discovered an unexpected new favourite: fizzy prune juice – the same colour as her beloved cola drinks!

HYPERACTIVITY

Hyperactive children are often not aware of their bad behaviour, but it is necessary to discipline and control them for their own sake and for the sanity of others. It is very hard therefore to be loving and sympathetic to a hyperactive child, even though this may be what he needs! This is a desperate vicious circle where everyone becomes more and more exhausted.

The Food Addict's Diet can provide a way out, as we discovered during the trials.

Sandy: A hyperactive child

Sandy was ten years old when his parents approached me for advice. A friend of theirs had found the diet useful when she was overweight, and as it also cured her panic attacks she recommended the diet to them in the hope that it might calm Sandy too.

For ten years Sandy had shown frequent outbursts of terrible anger, biting tantrums and destructive behaviour. This, and the sleepless nights, had driven his mother to exhaustion. Even as a small baby he had cried incessantly, and when he was four years old the family doctor diagnosed him as hyperactive.

When Sandy was seven, his mother suffered a nervous collapse, and he was taken into care for two weeks. He destroyed a great many of his foster mother's possessions and refused to eat. After only five days the foster mother refused to keep him any longer, and he was sent home again where his behaviour did improve a little under threat of return. His behaviour eventually broke up his parents' marriage and his father left home. Sandy's father had little to do with him for he could not cope with Sandy's behaviour and would not take him out.

After six weeks on the plan we saw occasional glimpses of a new Sandy who was calm and affectionate. The link between his behaviour and his diet was at last established, but the behaviour problem was not completely solved. At home he was much calmer, but he was just as excitable and difficult at school or in the street.

Now that an explanation for Sandy's behaviour had been found, his mother began to take the issue further. She told her husband about this discovery and together they found an allergy specialist who suggested that a chemical allergy might also be at work: Sandy could be reacting to petrol fumes in the street or cleaning materials used at school. These chemicals cannot be easily avoided, but the Food Addict's Diet and a course of vitamin and minerals prescribed by the allergy specialist to build up Sandy's general health have helped significantly. We now know that he becomes very irritable when given any of the four zeros, plus orange and tomato.

Sandy is now at secondary school, much happier and better behaved. The years of poor concentration have set him back in his studies but he is now making excellent progress for, like many hyperactive children, he is highly intelligent. He is showing a talent at woodwork, for now he can concentrate for long enough to finish his work properly, and made a spatula that won a class prize. Sandy gave his father the spatula for his Christmas present that year, and recently there has been talk of his father coming home to stay.

Help your child to understand his addictions

Some foods will be hard for your child to resist, for he is addicted to his 'trigger foods' and will be sorely tempted to take some if they are offered to him. Simply tell him that the foods he craves seem to 'wind him up', and that he will be happier without them because Mummy and Daddy will not need to shout at him so much.

In time he will need little encouragement to leave them alone, because he will have learned the difference between feeling miserable, panicky and irritable with his trigger foods, and feeling calm, happy and well loved without them. Then he will be happy to refuse the food rather than risk another episode of punishments and unhappiness. Once he has learned that, you will have won.

TAKE YOUR PARTNERS

If you want to persuade other members of your family to try the experiment, just encourage them to try it just as an experiment, and the results should speak for themselves. If the results have been good for you, there may be no problem at all, but never underestimate the ways in which addictive cravings can create all kinds of resistance to the idea. It may take time and a great deal of patience, but you can do it, and here is a good example of how it can be done.

Martin: a victim of executive stress?

Before he tried the experiment, Martin was very hard to live with. He used to worry constantly about his work, lose his temper at unpredictable moments, and make the most out of every stressful situation. At the same time he was loving, affectionate and childishly anxious to please. People found him exhausting because of his driving nervous energy that drained both himself and all those around him.

He blamed his psychological problems on his childhood, which had been fraught with trauma and emotional upset. Both friends and psychologists told him that he could not change the past and must accept it, but he carried all his personal grievances, past and present, around with him as an outsized 'chip' on his shoulder.

How could the Food Addict's Diet help a person such as this? Well, it took time, a patient wife, a certain amount of secrecy, but we did it.

Martin put every kind of excuse in the way when the experiment was first suggested. He declared such a major diet change would be impossible with all those business lunches and his stressful existence!

Gradually and quietly, his wife made diet changes at home to reduce Martin's intake of bread and sugar, which were his principal weaknesses. His wife allowed the bread to run out from time to time, and they used rye crispbread instead. She made fruit salads for dessert instead of his favourite pies and puddings, began to use honey instead of sugar, and changed to decaffeinated coffee.

Martin did not notice the change at first, but within a month his wife said that he seemed to be less tired and smiled more often at his little daughter. His wife suggested to him then that this new healthy diet was helping, but he roared on, denying any possibility that the improvement could be in any way related to his diet. However, it had set him thinking. An intelligent man, Martin began to take an interest in nutrition, to the extent that his workmates thought that he was turning into a 'health freak', and began to treat the whole thing as a huge joke.

It is to his credit that Martin resisted this peer pressure. He had already started gathering information from books and magazines about the effects of food on mood, and he was secretly beginning to think that there might be something in it after all. He had already begun to notice that he was coping better with stress at work, but was reluctant to admit it at first.

Finally he agreed to try the four zero experiment. The first week put him to bed for two days with a splitting headache and diarrhoea, which were probably withdrawal symptoms. Martin is a cautious man when it comes to his health, and so consulted his doctor, who found nothing wrong.

He told me that the next ten days were like 'climbing out of a quicksand': he wanted to climb out, but his love of Danish pastries, sugary food and red wine pulled him back. I reassured him that this was the effect of addiction, and to overcome it he had only to stick to the diet and wait. As time went by every new day was easier, and by the end of the second week his wife described him as 'human again', and he still is.

Now, a year later, he has lost a stone in weight, sleeps better, and finds that the stiffness in his ankle joints that he had put down to a lack of exercise has eased. He has taken up badminton again because it no longer hurts him to play. The pain in his joints has become a kind of barometer for his progress on the diet: when he lapses by taking his beloved pastries and red wine the pain returns to remind him of his mistake.

SPREADING THE WORD

People who try the experiment become imbued with an infectious enthusiasm for their new diet, and backed up by improvements in their health they make excellent evangelists; but many of them have told me how hard it is to persuade their friends and family to try it, owing to the resistance created by their food addictions.

I hope this chapter has shown you how, with a little patience and a great deal of understanding based on your own experiences on the four zero plan, you can lead others to try it, just for a while. This diet is hard to appreciate by just reading a book like this, as you know already. The feelings the diet can give you are hard to describe to others, and the only way for them really to understand this is to follow the Food Addict's Diet for themselves.

CHAPTER 15
A Diet for Life?

The time comes eventually when you have to face it: there is not much chance that you will ever be able to eat the way you did before you tried the four zero experiment without all your problems returning. The final step to take in overcoming addictions (see pages 87–9) is to face this simple fact. As a result of their struggles with this diet, all the trials candidates came face to face with their addiction to food, and the uncomfortable idea that addiction is a problem for life.

THREE GROUPS OF GUINEA PIGS

Through this book you have met several of my hundred guinea pigs, and they fall into three groups.

THE REFUSERS

This was the group whose addictions were so strong that they refused to consider even trying the experiment. Perfectly reasonable behaviour you might think, until you consider the nature of what they had to do: all I asked was for them to live without four food ingredients for three weeks, and I placed no restrictions whatsoever on how much they could eat. They were keen and anxious to try this 'new wonder diet', but only until they heard what was involved!

When I witnessed at first hand this total refusal to follow a diet that was totally unrestricted except for four vital ingredients, I began to realise that food addiction wars far more widespread than had been suggested in any of the books I had read about food intolerance.

I received several apologetic letters explaining why these applicants did not feel they could participate. Some of the letters were written after much heart searching, for they knew that a great deal was being asked of them by this simple set of rules, and they had to admit that they were not equal to the task.

The reasons were various, but boiled down to the same thing: food addiction. Either they thought that following the plan would require a complete change of lifestyle, or that giving up the zero foods was just too difficult, too expensive, or too inconvenient. Most of them bridled at the very idea that they were being described as 'food addicts'. Addicts in their view were weak-minded individuals who couldn't control themselves, and they wanted nothing to do with all that!

Perhaps this was once your view, or perhaps you have read this far and not yet tried the diet for precisely these reasons. You should have discovered by now that the zero plan does not require a change of lifestyle, and it is not expensive or inconvenient once you have made the first adjustments, which usually take about a week. As for addicts being considered 'weak-minded', that will be dealt with in further detail on page 237.

Some of this group did at last have a try at following the plan after some gentle persuasion, and they learned how their addiction had once moulded their view of food and their attitude to this diet as well. I was interested to see that one of my most adamant refusers, once he tried the diet, found it unexpectedly easy after all. Moreover, he did have a great deal of support from his wife, who had successfully lost a few pounds on the diet six months before and was well versed on how to make it inexpensive, interesting and satisfying. Even so, he was heard not long ago defending healthy eating among his peers at work, which has astonished everyone, including him!

THE SCEPTICS

The second group tried to treat the experiment simply as an experiment, and were anxious to keep their scepticism intact throughout, little knowing how far-reaching the effects of this diet change would be. They doubted my ideas from the start, and saw the whole thing as a challenge and 'just a piece of research'.

Although this group may appear negative when described in this way, I valued their findings very highly indeed, because they were determined not to be swept along on a wave of unrealistic enthusiasm, and demanded clear explanations of exactly why they must give up these four foods, exactly why they had not lost weight despite depriving themselves of their favourites for so long, etc. After the experiment they were at pains to find the results insufficient considering all that deprivation, and some of them were even reluctant to admit that their symptoms had improved!

For instance, Deborah, whom you met on page 71, protested at the end of her three weeks on the zero plan that it had done nothing for the pains in her feet and ankles, which was the principal reason why she had tried it in the first place, even though she had lost twelve pounds in weight. A few days later she mentioned in passing that her requirement for pain killers had been reduced by half, and much later she admitted that eating wheat and milk products greatly increased the pain.

I took the results from this group very seriously indeed, for their positive statements were not made lightly, but dragged reluctantly from people who wanted to believe that they were not true. Deborah now can see that she was made sceptical by her addiction: she did not want to believe that wheat and milk, her strongest addictions, aggravated her arthritis. So far she has managed very well without both wheat and milk, remains slim, and is in far less pain than before she began the experiment.

Long-term follow-up studies revealed that all of this group had lapsed back into their old way of eating, as may be expected, as they did not have the benefit of this book or the national network of 'Winners' Groups (see page 301) to back them up. I eventually was able to talk to some of them about their feelings. Some of them had not lost weight on the diet and had thought of the experiment purely in terms of weight loss. They thought that they had failed both themselves and me, but of course they had misunderstood the idea of the experiment. This sense of failure had made them defiant and resistant to the whole idea, but I hope you have not made the same mistake.

Those who did lose weight on the experiment had gradually returned to their old eating habits after the experiment, and of course they saw their weight increase and their symptoms return. Even so, they expressed a desire to try again in the follow-up questionnaires. Many of them had tried to begin again repeatedly, but they couldn't get into the frame of mind to make a new beginning. They longed to feel again how they did during the experiment and taste that magic again.

I was able to provide back-up for some of them to begin again, and we discovered an interesting new slant: all of them were eating the four zeros again, but clearly some of their new shopping and eating habits still remained. Beginning again was just like putting on a familiar suit of clothes, and in less than a week the battle was won for each of them.

THE DIE-HARDS

Most of the case histories I have mentioned in previous chapters are from the third group: the stalwart die-hards. They entered into the whole project with enthusiasm, and reaped huge rewards as a result, even though some of them found it very difficult. They continued after the experiment was over and carried on with a modified form of the diet to solve their particular problems, adding greatly to the fund of knowledge I needed to complete this book.

The most confirmed addicts needed the greatest support, but those who gained the most reward were not always the least addicted. I have explained the refusal and scepticism of the other groups in terms of their addiction, but many of this third and most successful group were strongly addicted too. However, they always managed to keep a positive attitude to their addiction, and instead of giving up if they lapsed from the diet, they just began again as many times as it took, which illustrates very well the importance of keeping a positive attitude throughout.

This diet is slow and gentle and there are few dramatic moments after the fifth day, but this group did not give up for lack of quick results. They were willing to take notice of small improvements and changes and rejoice in them, adding all the tiny pieces of progress together to make a whole, even when things were not going very well.

Some of them thought initially that they were only addicted to one zero food, such as sugar, but soon discovered several other addictions subtly guiding them to other delights such as cheese (milk) or digestive biscuits (wheat). A few unfortunate members of this group were addicted to all four foods, and a few more besides. This small group of people, who of course represent many thousands of people nationwide, will have to avoid the four zero foods for a very long time, for food intolerance and the symptoms that accompany it can fade in time, but food addictions are for life.

A DIET FOR LIFE

Making the four zero plan your diet for life is not easy, because our staple foods have crept into every packet of food we buy and turn up on every plate at every meal. There are three main areas of difficulty: shopping, eating out and, that old chestnut, peer pressure.

SHOPPING

When you first started the experiment I expect that your greatest problem was getting hold of the ingredients you needed. In small villages, where the local shop stocks only a few lines, this is particularly difficult, and the best answer is to grow your own and use mail-order firms (see addresses on page 297). Urban-dwellers have the advantage here: they have access to sophisticated supermarkets, catering for a wide range of tastes and diet, and inexpensive street markets to supply those all-important fruits and vegetables.

Another problem is expense, because foods such as rye flour are regarded as specialist products by most supermarkets and only a few shops sell them, and then usually at an inflated price. Nevertheless, at least in the area where I live in Hertfordshire, it is clear that public demand can create enormous changes in food availability.

When I first came to live in Hertfordshire ten years ago, 100 per cent rye bread was almost unobtainable, but it became available on order about four years ago, and these days it is freely available every day on the shelves of a local chain of bakery shops. Clearly, this change was brought about by an increased demand for rye bread as more and more people found as a result of an allergy test that their symptoms were caused by wheat.

Public demand

The food industry generally is so sensitive to changes in public demand that I can see all kinds of substitute foods, such as sugar-free soya and almond milk, milk-free margarine and wheat-free slimmers' meals becoming more widely available, even in those little country shops: this diet can only become easier to follow

238

as we demand the foods we need to remain well.

Meanwhile, you can do your bit by asking for less usual foods wherever you go. If a food is not available where you shop, ask for it repeatedly by name. If you persist sufficiently, your wish will be granted, for good shopkeepers are there to serve *you*, not the food industry.

EATING OUT

People who are dependent upon public eating places for their food often have great difficulty sticking to an elimination diet such as the four zero plan. They are forced to patronise the Asian and Oriental eating places in order to have any choice of dishes at all. You may be able to change things if you ask for what you want wherever you go: if you buy sandwiches, try asking for crispbread sandwiches instead of bread, and if you are tired of eternal ham salads in the pub because all there is on the menu is sandwiches or rolls, then try asking if there is an alternative, explaining that you can't take bread. If the pub serves hot meals, ask your landlord for rice with your meat course in place of chips and a fresh fruit salad instead of ice cream or pie. If enough people begin to ask for this kind of food these alternatives may begin to appear regularly on pub menus, so keep asking.

Consider the early days of vegetarianism when it was thought weird consciously to avoid meat. Today, being a vegetarian is considered quite acceptable, if not admirable, behaviour. The day when the problems of food intolerance will be accepted by people who cater for the general public is not so far away.

I hope that one day wheat-free, sugar-free, milk-free dishes and an alternative to the ubiquitous chip will one day become available in most public eating places, including schools and hospitals.

PEER PRESSURE

We have come a very long way together since you thought 'food addiction' was an outlandish theory and that food cravings were a purely psychological problem. Of course there is an important psychological dimension to any addiction, but food addiction is clearly a physical problem. It is greatly aggravated by social pressure, though, because however it begins, it is certainly maintained by the attitudes of others. Tony, our cigarette smoker from Chapter 5, found that he had to give up not only his cigarettes but his role as 'a smoker' among his friends, and he is not sure which was the most difficult.

'Would you like a cup of tea?'

We carefully keep each other's food addictions satisfied in the name of 'hospitality'. This is why we offer each other the kind of food that brings comfort, such as cups of sweet, milky tea or coffee (sugar, milk and caffeine), chocolate gâteau (sugar, milk, wheat and theobromine) and lasagne verde (wheat, milk, tomato and peppers).

One of the most difficult foods to avoid at first is tea and coffee, simply because refusing is so embarrassing. You must stand by while your hostess goes to elaborate lengths to seek out an alternative, and you vow that you will never refuse tea again! It takes courage to drink a glass of water instead, or present your own tea bag or sachet of decaffeinated coffee, but happily this is becoming more acceptable as more people find they feel better without caffeine drinks. In some enlightened households you may be offered the choice of a caffeine-free hot drink, and I was even offered decaffeinated coffee recently at a school fête!

'Just a little won't hurt!'

One of the principal causes of breakdown on the Food Addict's Diet is the food we are offered by our friends. It is almost always based on the four zero foods, and if we attempt to resist it our friends make a fuss and insist that 'a little won't hurt'.

Friends even seem to conspire to prevent you from slimming: if you lunch on a 250-calorie slimming meal that looks like a glass of milk and three biscuits or a small plate of curry with rice, nobody will comment on the small size of your meal. However, if you eat a 250-calorie meal of ham and mixed salad, your friends express wonder that you have managed to eat so little for lunch! They are even likely to force a few biscuits on you later as you have 'been so good', almost as if they cannot bear the thought of you being without your 'fix' for the day.

'What's for dinner?'

People who live alone can follow the Food Addict's Diet easily, but those who have families or other people to cook for are under a subtle pressure to create two different kinds of meal: one without the zero foods for themselves, and another to provide the daily fix of zeros for the family. Most mothers feel very guilty if they 'deny' their children their sugar or chips, even if they give them alternatives that are far healthier and just as tasty. They seem to be aware that they are not denying them food, but the pleasures of their fix.

'Can I join in?'

Familiarity, they say, breeds contempt. In the case of food addiction, familiarity breeds compliance. In a Winners' Group, beginning the Food Addict's Diet together, it does not take long to feel quite comfortable serving herbal teas and oatcakes with pâté instead of coffee and biscuits, and talking of withdrawal symptoms instead of the weather.

So join with your friends and create a Winners' Group; demand special foods in the shops; serve unusual dishes to your family so often that they become old favourites; introduce your friends to dishes free of the four zeros and see how much they notice, and offer them alternatives to tea or coffee and see how many of them accept.

It will not take long if you work at it. When the magic

of the Food Addict's Diet has begun to show in your face, figure and personality, those seemingly indifferent people around you will begin to wonder what they have been missing by refusing to listen to your ramblings about 'four zero foods'. Very soon now they will sidle up to you quietly and ask: 'Can I join in?' – and then you will know that you can start exerting the peer pressure on *them*!

FINALE

Four years ago this book was only a dream. I just knew that there was a large group of people who were over-weight, lacking in energy, and suffering from a series of minor ailments and, as a result, were unhappy.

Perhaps you have read this far and still feel unsure about making a start: it is much easier than you can ever imagine once you have got going. I hope that one day you too will try it, however intractable your problem might seem, and rediscover your natural appetite and all the other magic of the four zero plan. Then perhaps you will attempt one of the slimming options to lose weight. You might even carry on to find out which foods are causing your symptoms, beat your other addictions, and try the plan on the rest of the family. In any case, join a Winners' Group and make new friends who will support you all the way. Whatever you do, be sure that the Food Addict's Diet will bring you happiness, a new figure and a new lease of life.

Part Four
Recipes and
Further Information

Recipes

SUBSTITUTES FOR THE FOUR ZEROS

MILK

Almond milk or cream
(Nectina, a ready-to-use almond milk, can be ordered from your local health-food shop. Address for orders: Kerryredd Ltd, 250 Rosendale Road, London SE 24.)

How to make your own:
2 tsps/10 ml honey   *1 pt/570 ml water*
2 oz/50 g raw almonds

Put almonds into blender and grind them with a little water. Gradually mix the rest of the water and honey. Keep unused milk in fridge and blend again before using. Use for sauces, desserts, drinks and for moistening dry desserts or muesli. Use within three days.

Variations:
Almonds in apple juice
Pine nuts, water and honey
Coconut and pineapple juice
Cashews, orange, honey and cinnamon for a hot spiced 'milk' drink

Seed milk

Grind 2 oz/50 g sesame or sunflower seeds in a little water. Soak overnight. Grind again and dilute to taste. Add a little honey if preferred. Use to strengthen soups, moisten muesli, or pour over desserts.

Variations:
Sesame seeds, mineral water and honey
Sunflower seeds with a little honey and vanilla

WHEAT

Mixed-grain bread (makes one 1 lb/450 g loaf)

½ oz/15 g fresh yeast or 2 tsps dried yeast
½ tsp fructose
½ pt/275 ml hand-hot water
4 oz/100 g wholemeal barley flour
4 oz/100 g wholemeal rye flour
2 oz/50 g brown rice flour
3 oz/75 g fine-ground oatmeal
1 tsp salt
1 tbsp olive oil
1 tbsp poppy seeds

Dissolve yeast in water. (If using dried yeast, stir in fructose too and leave in a warm place for 10–15 minutes until frothy.) Combine the flours, oatmeal, salt and oil in a large bowl. Add the yeast liquid and mix to a dough. Knead 10 minutes, place in a bowl, cover, and leave until doubled in bulk (1 hour in a warm place). Knock back, knead briefly, shape and put into a greased 1 lb/450 g loaf tin. Sprinkle with poppy seeds. Cover and leave in a warm place until doubled in size. Bake loaf at 220°C/425°F/gas mark 7 for 10 minutes. Reduce heat to 200°C/400°F gas mark 6, for a further 20 minutes. Cool on a wire rack.

Quick rice bread

8 oz/225 g rice flour
½ tsp cream of tartar
2 tbsps olive oil
½ tsp salt
¼ pt/150 ml water

Pre-heat oven to 190°C/375°F/gas mark 5. Combine water and oil. Gradually stir into sifted dry ingredients. Bake in a greased 1 lb/450 g bread tin for about 30 minutes. Turn out on to a wire rack to cool. (From Robert Buist, *Food Intolerance and How to Cope with It.*)

Highland oatcakes (makes 8)

4 oz/100 g fine oatmeal	*3–4 tbsps hot water*
1 oz/25 g dripping or	*pinch of salt*
vegan margarine	*1 tsp bicarbonate of soda*
pinch of salt	

Melt fat with 3–4 tbsps water. Mix oatmeal, salt and bicarbonate of soda in a bowl. Make a well in the centre, pour fat and water mixture into the well, and knead into a dough. Make into eight small flat cakes. Place on a greased oven tray and bake in a moderate oven until browned at the edges. Cool on the tray and keep in an airtight tin. (From Catherine Brown, *Scottish Regional Recipes.*)

Non-wheat pastry (makes about 1 lb/450 g pastry)

2 oz/50 g barley flour	*2 oz/50 g vegan*
4 oz/100 g brown rice	*margarine*
flour	*2 oz/50 g lard*
2 oz/50 g cornflour	*pinch of salt*
1 tbsp fructose (for sweet	*cold water to mix*
pastry only)	

Sieve flour into a large bowl, incorporating as much air as you can. Rub in the fat until the mixture looks like fine breadcrumbs. Add water in small amounts until the mixture just begins to stick together. Turn on to a board sprinkled with cornflour and work the mixture into a round shape. Gather into a ball and chill in the fridge covered with foil or cling film for at least 30 minutes. Place on a board and roll out evenly, lightly and gently.

Bake as required at 200°C/400°F/gas mark 6 for about 20 minutes or until lightly browned.

NOTE: Try various combinations of non-wheat flours until you find a mixture that you like, but I find that the one above works the best.

SUGAR

Date purée
6 oz/175 g stoned fresh   orange juice
*   or dried dates, chopped*

Place dates in a small saucepan and add enough orange juice to cover. Simmer until mushy, adding a little more orange juice if necessary. Liquidise or mash until smooth. Use as a sweetener for cooked fruit or in place of sugar in fruit cake (see page 284).

POTATOES

Baked sweet potatoes (serves 4 as an accompaniment)
2 large sweet potatoes   seasoning
a little olive oil and salt
milk-free margarine to
*   serve*

Scrub skins of the potatoes thoroughly, remove damaged areas or blemishes, but do not peel. Cut into 3–4 oz/ 75–100 g pieces. Brush with a little oil and salt. Bake in a fairly hot oven (200°C/400°F/gas mark 6) for about 40 minutes, or until soft. After cooking, cut open and add a knob of milk-free margarine and seasoning if desired.

Variation:
For a quicker recipe, the prepared potatoes can be started off in a microwave for 3 minutes before baking in the oven, or they can be cooked entirely in a microwave for about 9 minutes.

Parsnip chips (serves 4 in place of potato chips)

2 large parsnips, peeled and cut into sticks	*3–4 tbsps olive oil*

Parboil parsnips for about 5 minutes in rapidly boiling water. Drain well on kitchen paper. Heat the oil in a heavy-based frying pan and when the oil is very hot (but *not* smoking!), quickly shallow-fry parsnip pieces, turning often. When browned, transfer chips carefully with a fish-slice or spatula on to kitchen paper. Keep hot and serve as soon as possible.

NOTE: These chips tend to be rather soggy. The trick is to make sure you do not boil them for too long before frying, and then fry them quickly in hot oil.

Variation:
Try this with sweet potatoes.

SAVOURY SPREADS

1. Try high-protein spreads such as tahini, hummus, or sunflower spread on crispbreads or rye bread – these are obtainable from health-food shops.
   2. Patum Peperium will blow your socks off, but do try it – carefully! If you like it, make your own with canned anchovies.

Nut butter

shelled nuts, such as
  peanuts, cashews,
  hazelnuts, etc.

a little olive oil
honey or fructose to taste

Grind any shelled nut finely in a blender, adding a little oil to make a spreading consistency. Sweeten with a little honey or fructose to taste. Add carob or vanilla for extra flavour.

SWEET SPREADS

Try pear and apple spread, or sugar-free jams, available from good supermarkets or health-food shops.

Apricot spread

8 oz/225 g apricots

¼ pt/150 ml apple juice

Soak apricots overnight, then simmer in apple juice for 30 minutes. Blend into a purée. Chill.

Apple and cinnamon spread

2 large dessert apples
4 oz/100 g fresh dates (if
  only dried dates are
  available, soak
  overnight in ½ pt/250 ml
  apple juice or water)

a pinch of cinnamon

Peel apples and stone dates. (Drain apple juice from soaked dry dates and use for a drink.) Purée in a food processor. Add cinnamon to taste.

DRINKS

Hot drinks

1. Take any pure juice, add a sweetener (honey, date purée, maple syrup), a few spices (cinnamon, mixed spice) and some hot water, and then mix to taste.

2. Put two slices of lemon in a mug. Add honey to taste and boiling water. Sip slowly. Add a herb tea bag with camomile for an extra-soothing cuppa.

3. Add carob to soya milk and heat gently, and sweeten with maple syrup. This makes a good cocoa substitute.

4. Heat up left-over vegetable juice, add a little vegetable stock paste and stir well. Good for very cold days or if you are very tired.

5. Try every one of the herb teas, including the combined-flavour teas. There will be at least one of them you like!

Cold drinks

1. Try mixing apple juice or orange juice with fizzy mineral water for a refreshing cold drink.

2. Mix pure pineapple juice, pure orange juice, a dash of lemon juice, fizzy mineral water and crushed ice. Drink through the ice with a straw. Add coconut milk for a nutritious cocktail.

BREAKFASTS

Apple sunrise (serves 1–2)

1 large dessert apple, washed	2 fresh dates (or 1 tbsp dried and chopped)
2 tsps crushed hazelnuts/ almonds/walnuts	1 tsp desiccated coconut
2 tsps sunflower seeds	¼ pt/150 ml fresh orange juice

Grate the apple. Top with crushed nuts, sunflower seeds, dates and coconut. Pour orange juice over. Eat at once. (From Robert Buist, *Food Intolerance and How to Cope with It*.)

Buckwheat pancakes (makes 6 pancakes)

2 oz/50 g buckwheat
  flour
2 oz/50 g wholemeal
  barley or rye flour
pinch salt

1 egg
a little olive oil
1 tbsp maple syrup
1 tbsp lemon juice

Put buckwheat flour, barley or rye flour, salt and egg into a blender and mix for 1–2 minutes. Leave to stand for about 10 minutes. Add oil to a small frying pan. Heat until beginning to smoke. Add enough mixture to cover bottom of pan. Turn carefully after about 2 minutes and brown other side. Mix maple syrup with lemon juice in a small jug and pour a little over each pancake. Fold in halves or quarters. Serve at once.

Dried fruit compôte

Equal quantities of:
    dried apricots
    prunes
    dried pears
    dried apples
¼ pt/150 ml orange juice
water
cinnamon to taste

Soak fruit overnight. The next day put into a large pan, add orange juice and enough water to cover the fruit. Add some raisins and a little cinnamon or honey to taste. Simmer for 15 minutes. Cool before eating.

This is delicious with left-over rice as breakfast. I recommend making enough for several days as this keeps well in the fridge.

Kidney and pease pudding breakfast (serves 1)

1 small onion   *olive oil*
1 lamb's kidney
2 tbsps pease pudding
  (see below)

Fry onion gently until brown. Slice kidney and put into pan beside onion, and fry gently for 2 or 3 minutes, turning often. Add pease pudding to the pan. Cover and cook over gentle heat for a further 5 minutes.

Muesli

Choose from the following groups of foods according to your taste:

1. *Cereals*: barley flakes, rye flakes, oat flakes, millet flakes, soya flakes. Soak in fruit juice overnight.
2. *Seeds*: sunflower, flax, sesame, melon, pumpkin. Crush or grind, mix with soaked cereal just before eating.
3. *Dried fruit*: raisins, apricots, apple, pineapple, pear, peach. Soak overnight in water or cook for a hot muesli.
4. *Nuts*: peanuts, pine nuts, hazelnuts, walnuts (ground or chopped). Sprinkle over muesli mixture and eat at once.
5. *Fresh fruit*: apple, banana, pear, peach, orange, melon or soft fruit. Chop roughly and add to muesli just before eating.

NOTE: If you forget to soak ingredients, cook cereals and dried fruits in fruit juice for a few minutes and eat hot, adding any other ingredients just before serving.

Pease pudding (serves 4)

8 oz/225 g yellow split   *1 tbsp olive oil*
  peas   *salt and pepper*
1 large onion

Put peas in a saucepan with a good covering of cold water. Bring to the boil and simmer until tender and mushy (can take 30 minutes to 1 hour). Drain off excess water. Peel and chop onion and fry gently in oil until soft. Add onion to cooked peas and season. This cooked mixture keeps well in the fridge for a quick snack or even a sandwich filling! To vary, try adding lemon rind, chopped sage or a pinch of ground cloves.

Variation:
Add an egg to make a baked pease pudding. Bake in a moderate oven at 180°C/350°F/gas mark 4 for 30–40 minutes (serves 4).

Kedgeree (serves 4)

12 oz/350 g smoked haddock
6 oz/175 g long-grain rice
2 hard-boiled eggs
3 tbsps oil
salt
about ¼ tsp cayenne pepper
2 tbsps finely chopped fresh parsley (or 1 tbsp dried parsley)

Cook and flake fish. Cook rice in usual way. Chop eggs. (This can be done in advance.) Put oil in saucepan and add the fish, egg and parsley; mix gently and add salt and cayenne to taste. Stir over a moderate heat for 5 minutes. Serve at once.

Porridge (serves 2)

4 oz/100 g medium-ground oatmeal, conservation grade rolled oats or quick-cook oat flakes
½ pt/275 ml fruit juice
½ pt/275 ml water
1 ripe banana, mashed
cinnamon to taste

Soak oats overnight in fruit juice. Place in heavy-based saucepan and add water. Cook as slowly as you can over a gentle heat for 15–20 minutes or a little longer. Remove from heat and add mashed banana. Sprinkle with cinnamon if desired, and serve at once.

Alternatives for oatmeal porridge:
1. Rice: mix left-over rice with prunes: delicious!
2. Cook oat and barley flakes together and sweeten with honey.
3. Soak millet flakes, buckwheat (kasha) or sago overnight and cook as porridge.

Scrambled eggs (serves 1)

2 eggs	salt and pepper
1 tbsp olive oil	
2 tbsps of almond milk (see page 245)	

Heat oil in a saucepan. Add almond milk and bring slowly to boil. Mix eggs in a cup and add seasoning. Pour into saucepan, stirring vigorously with a wooden spoon. When the eggs begin to set, remove from heat and continue stirring. Pour on to rice cakes spread with vegan margarine.

Super muesli (serves 4)

2 oz/50 g dates	1 oz/25 g ground hazelnuts
3 oz/75 g dried apricots	2 tbsps dried coconut
1 banana	2 oz/50 g raisins
1 oz/25 g rolled oats	1 tsp cinnamon
1 oz/25 g barley flakes	apple juice to soak
1 oz/25 g rye flakes	

Chop dried fruit, grind nuts, slice banana. Mix well with cinnamon and other dry ingredients. Leave to soak overnight in apple juice.

LUNCHES

Chicken liver pâté (serves 4–6)

8 oz/225 g chicken livers
2 medium onions,
   roughly chopped
2 cloves garlic, chopped
a little olive oil
1 tbsp lemon juice

salt and pepper
1 tbsp mayonnaise or
   1 oz/25 g vegan
margarine (to soften if
   required)

Braise onion and garlic and chicken livers in a little oil.
Cover and leave to simmer for about 25 minutes. Purée
in a processor. Add lemon juice and seasoning to taste.
Press into a shallow dish and chill in the fridge. If too
dry, add a little mayonnaise or vegan margarine, mix
well, and chill again before serving.

Mackerel pâté (serves 4–6)

12 oz/350 g skinned,
   boned smoked
   mackerel

1 tbsp mayonnaise
1 tbsp horseradish sauce

Purée all ingredients in a food processor for about 20
seconds. Press into a small shallow dish. Chill. Serve
with oatcakes or rye crispbread, cucumber slices and
celery sticks.

Pork and liver pâté (serves 4)

8 oz/225 g pork offcuts,
   chopped
4 oz/100 g chicken livers,
   chopped
1 large or two small
   onions, chopped

3 cloves garlic, crushed
2 tbsps olive oil for frying
mayonnaise to mix
salt and pepper
mixed herbs

Fry chopped pork offcuts and chicken livers in a heavy-
based pan with garlic and onion for about 5 minutes.
Leave covered to simmer for about 40 minutes. Put into
a food processor and mix for a few seconds. (If you do

256

not have a food processor, allow to cool and then mince finely.) Chill in the fridge overnight. When cold, put into a bowl and add enough mayonnaise to make a soft spreading consistency. Add salt, pepper and mixed herbs to taste. Serve with crispbreads or rye toast.

Sardine salad (serves 2–3)
Drain a can of sardines (in brine) carefully and coat with mayonnaise. Lay on a bed of lettuce and garnish with parsley. Add sliced hard-boiled egg as a variation.

NOTE: If using sardines in olive oil, reserve the oil for frying other fish.

Squeak-and-bubble (serves 1–2)

8 oz/225 g left-over vegetables (carrots, parsnip, greens, peas, etc.) cooked and mashed

1 onion, finely chopped
1 tbsp olive oil
1 tbsp cornflour
1 egg

Mix vegetables together with cornflour. Fry onion in olive oil, add vegetables and form into a flat cake. Allow to char slightly before turning. Top with a poached egg.

PACKED LUNCHES

Choose one from each of these six sets of ingredients for maximum variety. Wrap food in greaseproof paper. (Plastic film can cause reactions and is not bio-degradable.)

Crispbreads
Rye crispbreads (Ryvita, Scanda Crisp, Finncrisp) or rice cakes.

Non-wheat bread
Rye, barley or mixed-grain bread (see page 246).

Protein
Small pieces of cooked meat; nuts or seeds; cold cooked fish; hummus; nut butters or seed spreads (see pages 249–50); pâtés made from liver, pork, chicken, vegetables or fish (see page 256).

Vegetables
Crudités (see below); salads made from raw or cold cooked vegetables tossed in French dressing or mayonnaise.

Fruit
Any kind.

Sweet treats
Biscuits or scones made using other flours; small packs of mixed dried tropical fruit, nuts and seeds.

STARTERS

Crudités
broccoli spears, broken into small pieces
cucumber, cut into sticks
carrot, cut into thin sticks
celery sticks, cut in half

Arrange in a flat dish in groups around a small dish full of some kind of dip (see below). Take pieces in your fingers and dip them into the dip. (Makes a useful starter for a buffet meal.)

Cashew dip (serves 4)
4 oz/100 g cashews
¼ pt/150 ml water
2 cloves garlic, finely chopped
2 tbsps lemon juice
3 spring onions, finely chopped
1–2 tbsps vegetable stock (if required)

Blend together in a food processor or blender. Add enough vegetable stock to make desired consistency. Chill and serve. Will keep for four days in the fridge. (Recipe provided by Mrs J. C., a 1987 trials candidate.)

Guacamole (serves 4)

1 ripe, soft avocado
1 clove garlic, crushed

2 tbsps lemon juice
salt and pepper to taste

Remove flesh from avocado. Put into a liquidiser with remaining ingredients. Chill. Serve with corn chips and crudités.

Lentil and vegetable soup (serves 4–6)

6 oz/175 g red lentils
1½ pts/840 ml vegetable stock or juices (see page 270)
1 medium onion, finely chopped

1 tbsp olive oil
2 sticks celery, sliced
3 medium carrots, roughly chopped
salt and pepper

Put lentils into a saucepan with the stock and bring to the boil. Simmer until the lentils begin to soften (about 10 minutes). Meanwhile, fry onion in a little olive oil for about 5 minutes. Add the celery and carrot and stir-fry for a further 5 minutes. Add to lentils and bring to the boil. Turn down heat and simmer until all the ingredients are very soft. Season to taste. If you like a smooth soup, liquidise or sieve for a few seconds.

Prawn (shrimps) and melon (serves 4)

1 honeydew or ogen melon
4 oz/100 g shrimps or prawns, cooked and cooled

mayonnaise (see page 267)

Cut melon into bite-sized pieces, or make balls with a melon-baller or small spoon. Add to prepared prawns/

shrimps and mix together. Divide into four portions and place a tablespoon of mayonnaise on each.

Small fried fish (serves 4)

12 oz/350 g fresh or
  frozen whitebait, sprats
  or sardines, headed,
  cleaned and gutted
2–4 tbsps olive oil (either
  fresh or reserved from
  a can of sardines)

3 tbsps cornflour, barley
  flour or very finely
  ground oats (see note
  below)

Prepare whole fish by removing heads and guts, or buy ready-prepared. Toss all the fish together in the flour in a bowl and shallow fry in oil, turning frequently. Add more oil if required. Drain in crumpled kitchen paper. Serve with a quartered lemon and plenty of extra lemon juice.

NOTE: If you want to use oatmeal for this recipe, place fine-ground oatmeal or porridge oats in a grinder and grind into a powder. Spare oatmeal can be kept for another recipe.

Variation:
Serve cold on a bed of shredded lettuce and cucumber with French dressing (see page 266).

Celery soup (serves 4)

1 onion, chopped
1 oz/25 g lean bacon,
  chopped
1 small head of celery,
  chopped

1 tbsp corn or rice flour
½ pt/275 ml soya milk
vegetable juices (see
  recipe, page 270) if
  required

Chop bacon and onion and gently fry them together for about 10 minutes until very soft. Remove from heat, add chopped celery and flour. Mix well. Cook on a low heat, stirring all the time. Add milk slowly until mixture thickens. Add vegetable juices to thin mixture if required. Reserve a ½ pt/250 ml of the mixture and liquidise the rest. Add reserved mixture and serve with rye bread croutons.

Chicken broth (serves 4 as main meal)

chicken carcass (the
    remains of a roast
    chicken)
2 pt/840 ml water or
    vegetables juices (see
    page 270)
3 leeks

1 turnip
1 onion
3 sticks celery
salt and pepper
2 oz/50 g short-grain rice
chopped fresh parsley to
    garnish

Cover carcass with water in a large pan and bring to the boil. Simmer for one hour or until the bones are getting soft. Remove the bones and fatty skin. Chill remaining stock overnight and remove fat, which will have formed a solid layer on top. Coarsely chop vegetables and place them in a large saucepan with the chicken stock. Season to taste. Add rice and simmer until rice is soft. Sprinkle parsley over each bowl to serve. (From *The Constance Spry Cookery Book*.)

Kale winter warmer (serves 4)

1 lb/450 g cheap beef or
    beef bones, trimmed of
    fat
2 oz/50 g pot barley

water or vegetable juices
    (see page 270)
8 oz/225 g kale

Simmer the beef or bones with the barley in enough water or vegetable juices to cover for 2–3 hours. Check water levels frequently and add more as necessary. Add kale 20 minutes before the end of the cooking time. Remove beef and bones before serving. Use beef for another meal. Serve in big, shallow bowls with rough pieces of mixed-grain bread (see page 246). (From Catharine Brown, *Scottish Regional Recipes*.)

Mushroom and barley miso soup (serves 4)

1 tbsp olive oil
1 onion, chopped
12 oz/350 g mushrooms,
 finely chopped
1 tsp thyme
1 tbsp pot barley
2 pt/840 ml vegetable
 stock (see page 270)
1 tsp miso (this is
 fermented soya,
 available from health-
 food shops)

1 small clove garlic,
 crushed
salt
2 tbsps chopped fresh
 parsley as garnish

Fry onion in oil. Chop mushrooms roughly and add to pan. Fry gently for 3 minutes. Add thyme, barley and stock. Stir in miso and garlic. Cook over a low heat, or until barley is soft and mixture has thickened slightly (about 40 minutes). Season with salt and add parsley as a garnish on each bowl. (From Robert Buist, *Food Intolerance and How to Cope with It*.)

Pea and bacon soup (serves 2–3)

1 small onion, chopped
2 rashers back bacon
3 oz/75 g green peas

1 pt/570 ml vegetable
 stock (see page 270)

Chop two rashers of bacon into small pieces. Fry with an onion until soft. Add peas and vegetable stock and bring to the boil. Cook for 10 minutes. Liquidise or sieve half the mixture, add to the rest and heat briefly. Serve at once with rough chunks of rye bread.

MAIN COURSES

Braised pork chop (serves 4)

1 small chop per person,
    or half a larger one
1 onion
1 tbsp olive oil
1 clove of garlic
1 pt/570 ml of vegetable
    stock, either home-
    made (see page 270) or
    made from vegetable
    stock paste

2 medium carrots
2 sticks celery
4 oz/100 g mushrooms
2 tsps of cornflour
a little water
1 bouquet garni
salt and pepper

Fry chops in oil over a moderate heat until all sides are sealed. Remove from pan. Lower heat and fry onions in same pan until soft. Add stock and vegetables to onions. Mix cornflour with a little water in a small bowl and add to the mixture, stirring well until it thickens. Add chops to mixture and mix gently. Add bouquet garni. Season to taste. Bring to the boil and simmer for 1½ hours, or until meat is tender. Check that the mixture does not go dry: if it does, add more stock during cooking. (Cooking time can be reduced to 1 hour if meat is first marinaded in French dressing over-night to tenderise it.) Serve with green vegetables and rice.

NOTE: Diced pork meat can also be used for this recipe.

Chicken casserole (serves 4)

1 medium onion, sliced
4 chicken quarters,
    skinned
½ pt/275 ml dry cider
½ pt/275 ml vegetable
    stock (see page 270)

4 sticks of celery,
    chopped
2 oz/50 g mushrooms,
    sliced
½ tsp mixed herbs
salt and pepper

Fry onion until soft, add chicken pieces. Brown the meat, turning frequently. Add cider, vegetable juices and vegetables. Mix gently. Add herbs and season to taste. Simmer until the chicken is soft (about 40 minutes). Serve with brown rice and steamed green vegetables.

Lamb and barley hot pot (serves 4)

1 chump chop per person, or 2 loin chops or 4 oz/100 g of diced lamb or mutton
1 medium onion, sliced
2 large carrots, sliced
1 turnip, roughly chopped
1 medium parsnip, roughly chopped

6 oz/175 g swede
3 oz/75 g mushrooms
3 oz/75 g pearl barley
1 pt/570 ml of vegetable stock, home-made (see page 270) or made from vegetable stock paste
½ tsp rosemary
salt and pepper

Fry onions in a little olive oil. Add chops and turn until sealed on all sides. Add diced vegetables and enough stock to cover. Add barley, herbs and seasoning. Mix well. Bring to boil and bake in oven, 160°C/325°F/gas mark 3, for about 1½ hours. Add more stock during cooking if necessary. (From *The Constance Spry Cookery Book*.)

Rabbit and bacon casserole (serves 4)

1 onion, sliced
1 clove of garlic, crushed
2 tbsps olive oil
8 oz/225 g rabbit meat, diced
4 rashers streaky bacon, chopped
2 tbsps fine-ground oat-meal

3 carrots, chopped
15 oz/450 g tin of kidney beans
2 oz/50 g mushrooms
3 oz/75 g sliced green beans (if available)
1 pt/570 ml vegetable stock (see page 270)

Gently fry garlic and onion in olive oil until soft. Add diced rabbit meat and continue to fry gently, turning frequently. Add chopped bacon and fry for another few minutes. Remove from heat, add oatmeal and mix well. Add vegetables and mix well. Cover with vegetable stock and bring to the boil, stirring gently. Simmer for 1 hour on top of stove or bake in a moderate oven for about 1 hour.

Variation
Add a little sliced apple and a handful of raisins to the vegetables.

Shepherd's parsnip pie (serves 4)

Parsnip purée

2 large parsnips, diced and boiled	a little vegan margarine salt and pepper

Peel and chop parsnips and simmer covered in just enough water to cover for 30 minutes until very soft. Drain and reserve the juice for the meat base. Mash or purée. Add a little margarine and salt and pepper to taste.

Meat base

10 oz/275 g minced lamb or beef	1 cup peas ½ pt/275 ml of vegetable
1 medium onion, sliced	stock
2 carrots, grated	1 tsp rice flour
4 oz/100 g mushrooms, chopped	

Fry onion until soft. Add mince and fry, stirring often, until it turns brown. Add carrots, mushrooms and peas. Add rice flour and stir well. Add stock and stir again. (If a thinner sauce is preferred, use parsnip juices reserved from making the parsnip purée.) Cook over a low heat for 20 minutes. Turn into a shallow dish and cover with the parsnip purée. Dot with margarine and sprinkle with a little salt. Bake in a moderate oven (180°C/350°F/gas mark 4) for 30 minutes, or until beginning to brown on top.

Variation
Mix a purée of cooked butter beans with the parsnip as an alternative topping.

Fish omelette (serves 4)

6 oz/175 g fillet of white
  fish lightly poached
2 tbsps soy sauce
1 tsp honey
4 large eggs

2 tsps olive oil
juice of 1 lemon
salt and pepper
1 tbsp chopped fresh
  parsley

Set aside some shreds of cooked fish for a garnish. Liquidise the rest of the fish, soy sauce, honey and eggs. Grease a shallow 10 in/25 cm oven-proof dish with oil. Pour in mixture and bake uncovered for about 40 minutes at 150°C/300°F/gas mark 2, until egg is set. Squeeze lemon juice over each serving and add some fresh parsley and a few shreds of fish. (Adapted from Jeremy Round, *The Independent Cook*.)

SALAD DRESSINGS

NOTE: Always toss salad in some kind of dressing, as the acid helps to preserve the natural enzymes raw vegetables contain.

French dressing

6 tbsps olive oil
3 tbsps wine or cider
  vinegar

salt and pepper

Shake all ingredients in a screwtop jar till well blended. Store in the fridge till needed.

NOTE: When tossing a green salad, first wipe the bowl with a cut clove of garlic, add some dressing to the empty bowl, then put in the salad and stir with two servers until the leaves are well covered. Tip the bowl to pour off any surplus dressing.

Vinaigrette

3 tbsps white wine vinegar or lemon juice
6 tbsps of olive oil
½ tsp of ready-made mustard (or ¼ tsp mustard powder)

2 tsps of chopped fresh mixed herbs, such as parsley, tarragon or mint (or ½ tsp of dried mixed herbs)
salt and pepper to taste

Shake in a screwtop jar and use as for French dressing.

NOTE: This makes a good marinade for meat before grilling.

Mayonnaise (with liquidiser)

1 whole egg
½ tsp of dry mustard
Salt and pepper

2 tsps vinegar
2 tsps lemon juice
7 fl oz/200 ml olive oil

Break egg into liquidiser and add salt, pepper, vinegar and lemon juice. Blend for 1 minute at medium speed. Then turn speed up high and gradually add the oil, drop by drop through the hole in the lid of the goblet. When you have added about half the oil, the sound will change as the mixture thickens. At that stage you can add the rest of the oil slowly in a thin stream. If the mayonnaise is a bit thick, add some boiling water to thin it a little.

NOTE: Persevere with this recipe until you get it right: you will not regret it, because home-made mayonnaise is far superior to any you can buy.

SALADS

Mayonnaise salad (serves 4)

8 oz/225 g left-over
  cooked vegetables, e.g.
  carrots, French beans,
  parsnips
2 sticks of celery, sliced
1 dessert apple, diced
mayonnaise to mix (see
  page 267)
1 hard-boiled egg,
  chopped
fresh parsley, finely
  chopped
a little paprika pepper

Mix all ingredients gently, adding enough mayonnaise to
bind. Sprinkle with fresh parsley and a little paprika
pepper if desired.

NOTE: Paprika is a nightshade (see pages 37–8).

Chewy Salad (serves 4)

1 tbsp pine nuts
2 tbsps orange juice
Choose at least four of the following:
  white cabbage, grated
  carrot, grated
  cooking apple, grated
  celery, chopped
  mushrooms, peeled and sliced thinly
  raw beetroot, peeled and sliced
  watercress

Place chosen vegetables and nuts in a large bowl. Add
orange juice. Toss well. Toss again before serving.

Crunchy salad (serves 4)

1 tbsp sunflower seeds
2 tbsps French dressing (see page 266)
Choose at least four of the following:
  celery, chopped
  iceberg lettuce, shredded

radishes, sliced
cucumber, sliced
carrots, sliced
chicory
Chinese leaves

Tasty Salad (serves 4)
1 tbsp sesame seeds
2 tbsps vinaigrette dressing (see page 267)
Choose at least four of the following:
watercress
rape and cress
cos or Webb's lettuce
chives
spring onion
Spanish onion
bean sprouts
radishes
dandelion leaves
geranium leaves

VEGETABLES

Exotic vegetables and how to prepare them

Fennel
Grate into a salad; cook for soup; braise as a side dish.

Jerusalem artichokes
Serve grated or sliced raw in salads.

Sweet potato
Roast with meat or with other whole vegetables. Try adding dill seeds for flavour.

Salsify
Slice into lemon juice and add to salad, or fry in a little oil.

Nettles
Simmer until soft and serve as you would spinach, or add to soup.

Radish tops/beetroot tops/turnip tops
Stir fry in oil or cook as you would spinach.

Vegetable stock
Simply strain off the cooking water from any cooked vegetables, pour into a jug, and keep in the fridge and use in place of stock in soups and casseroles. Use within two or three days.

VEGETARIAN DISHES

While you are avoiding milk, your protein base will be wholegrains, seeds, beans, peas and pulses if you are vegan, plus eggs or even fish if you simply avoid meat. These recipes are for those who eschew all animal protein.

COOKING HINTS

Wholegrains

Rye grains
Method: soak overnight, keeping grains covered. Bring to the boil and simmer in a covered pan. Cook for about 1 hour, until grains burst.

Whole rye is also available as flakes and 100 per cent wholemeal flour.

Brown rice
Method: wash grains thoroughly. Using twice as much water as rice, bring to boil and simmer in a covered pan for 20–30 minutes until all water is absorbed.

Brown rice is also available as brown rice flour. Do not use white rice, rice flakes or ground rice unless you have no alternative, as white rice is less nourishing, having lost most of its B vitamins and minerals when polished.

Millet
No need to soak. Using three times as much water as millet, bring to the boil and cook in a covered pan for 15 minutes, stirring when necessary. You can add a little extra flavour by dry-roasting the grains for a few minutes before adding water.

Millet is also available as flakes.

Pot barley
Soak overnight in three times the volume of water. The next day bring to the boil. Cover and simmer for at least 2 or 3 hours, until soft.

Pearl barley
No need to soak. Using enough water to keep grains covered throughout, bring to boil and simmer for 1–2 hours, until soft.

NOTE: Pearl barley is not as nutritious as pot barley as most of the goodness is in the outer skin which is polished off during processing.

Buckwheat
No need to soak. Dry-roast the grains for a few minutes by heating in a heavy-based pan, stirring continuously. Add twice the volume of water, bring to the boil and cook for 10–20 minutes or until soft.

Buckwheat is also available as flour, noodles and kasha (roasted buckwheat).

Pulses

Slow-cook varieties
These are butter beans, kidney beans, soya beans, chick-peas, black beans and dried broad beans.

Soak beans overnight. Drain them and put into a pan

271

with twice the volume of fresh water. Bring to the boil for a few minutes and then simmer covered until soft, about 40–60 minutes. A bay leaf adds flavour. Do not add salt as this makes them tough.

Bulk-cook these in advance and freeze. They will keep in the fridge for a week.

IMPORTANT NOTE: When cooking kidney beans, first boil rapidly *for at least 10 minutes*, as they contain toxins that are not destroyed by simmering. Never cook raw kidney beans in a 'slow-cooker': use canned beans instead.

Quicker-cooking varieties
These are black-eyed beans, aduki beans, dried whole green peas, haricot beans and flageolets.

Soak overnight before cooking or, if short of time, bring to boil and set aside in their water for 1 hour. Drain, bring to the boil again in fresh water and simmer for about 45 minutes.

Quick-cook pulses
These are green lentils, yellow split peas, red lentils and mung beans.

Soaking overnight reduces cooking time, but all these can be cooked without soaking. Bring to the boil in enough water to cover and simmer for 20–30 minutes.

Experiment with this group by adding any of them raw to casseroles or soups before cooking with the other ingredients. They will add extra cheap protein and bulk to any savoury dish.

Bean salad
(When using canned beans, strain and rinse off the sugar first)

Choose at least 4 of the following canned beans, strained and rinsed:

kidney beans
flageolet beans
broad beans
haricot beans
green beans, cooked and cooled
garden peas, cooked and cooled
1 onion, chopped very finely
1 tbsp parsley, chopped finely
2 tbsps vinaigrette dressing

Toss all ingredients together in a large bowl. This is excellent as a main vegetarian dish with a green salad and rice, or as a filling vegetable with cold meat or fish. Particularly good with smoked mackerel.

Instant fried rice (serves 2 as main dish, 4 as an accompaniment)

1 large onion, roughly chopped
1 tbsp olive oil for frying
4 oz/100 g fresh or frozen peas

8 oz/225 g cooked brown rice
1 tbsp olive oil with rice
1–2 tbsps soy sauce (to taste)

Stir-fry onion until soft, about 5 minutes. Add the peas and stir-fry for a few more minutes. Add rice and mix well. Add more oil and stir-fry mixture until heated through. Sprinkle with soy sauce to taste and serve at once. (A recipe idea from one of my trial candidates.)

Variations
1. Add chopped left-over vegetables, canned sweetcorn, thinly sliced mushrooms or canned beans to mixture in place of peas.
2. Use any other left-over cooked whole grains with, or in place of, the rice.

Millet and vegetables (serves 2 as a main meal, 4 as an accompaniment)

4 oz/100 g millet grains
1 pt/570 ml vegetable
   stock or juices (see
   page 270) bouquet
   garni
1 tbsp olive oil
3 medium carrots, finely
   chopped

1 large parsnip, finely
   chopped
3 oz/75 g garden peas,
   fresh or frozen
2 oz/50 g mushrooms,
   sliced
salt and pepper

Simmer the millet in the vegetable stock with a bouquet garni until soft (about 15 minutes). Meanwhile, in a large saucepan, gently stir-fry finely chopped vegetables in a little sesame oil until soft (about 10 minutes). Remove bouquet garni from millet and add to onion. Mix vegetables into the millet and season to taste. (Adapted from a recipe suggestion on the back of the first packet of millet I ever bought in 1987.)

Mixed wholegrains (serves 4)

4 oz/100 g pot barley
3 oz/75 g millet
4 oz/100 g brown rice
4 oz/100 g canned sweet-
   corn

1½ pt/750 ml vegetable
   stock (see page 270)
bay leaf
salt and pepper
other seasoning as desired

Soak barley and millet overnight. Boil barley for 2 hours or until it is beginning to soften. Drain and put into a pan with vegetable stock and bay leaf. Add millet and rice and simmer covered for 20 minutes. Add the corn and mix carefully. Simmer uncovered until water is absorbed. Remove bay leaf and season with salt and pepper.

Experiment with other flavours and spices by adding a little to a small portion to find a suitable taste. Try curry powder, cayenne pepper, paprika pepper, celery salt or garlic salt.

This can be made in batches to freeze. Frozen mixture

can be stir-fried with garlic and chopped mixed vegetables for an instant meal. (Adapted from a recipe by Gail Duff in her book, *The Pick of the Crop*.)

Rice with lentils (serves 4)

8 oz/225 g brown lentils
  (soaked overnight if
  possible)
1 pt/570 ml water
3 medium onions,
  chopped
4 tbsps olive oil

8 oz/225 g brown rice,
  washed and drained
salt and pepper
8 oz/225 g spinach,
  washed
2 cloves of garlic, crushed
½ tsp all-spice

If they have been soaked overnight, drain lentils: otherwise rinse them. Place in a large saucepan with the water and allow to boil covered for 10 minutes. Fry one of the onions in 2 tablespoonfuls of the oil in another pan and add with the rice to the cooking lentils. Mix well. Cover and cook for 40 m nutes. Meanwhile, cook the spinach for about 10 minutes and drain well. Add to the cooked rice and lentils and mix together evenly. Season to taste.

Fry sliced onions in remaining oil until dark and add crushed garlic and all-spice. Cook for a few minutes, stirring slowly. Sprinkle this mixture on top of the rice/lentil/spinach mixture in a serving dish. Serve hot with green vegetables or cold with salad. (Adapted from an Indian recipe.)

RECIPES USING SEEDS

NOTE: Edible seeds of any kind (see page 102) can be bought from health-food shops. They can be added to any raw or cooked vegetable dish for extra flavour and goodness. The Romans used to use flax seed as a condiment on many of their savoury dishes, and so can you!

Vegetable stir-fry (serves 4)

2 tbsps sesame oil
1–2 cloves of garlic,
  crushed
1–2 onions, sliced thinly
1 lb/450 g mixed,
prepared vegetables (see
  below)

1 tbsp flax, sesame or
  sunflower seeds

Vegetable suggestions

parsnip: cut into thin
  sticks
celery: chop
mushroom: slice thinly
fennel: slice thinly, use
  sparingly
carrots: cut into thin
  sticks or slice very thin
  lengthways
mangetout peas: leave
  whole

Brussels sprouts: slice
  into rings
cabbage heart: shred well
broccoli spears: divide
  into tiny pieces
beansprouts: home-grown
  (see page 102) or
  purchased, washed and
  well drained

NOTE: Do not grate or use processor as this produces a mushy result.

Prepare vegetables immediately before cooking, and mix together in a large bowl. Crush the garlic and sauté in sesame oil with the onion in a large heavy-based pan, casserole dish or wok. Add vegetables to onion and garlic all at once. Toss the mixture with a wooden spoon over a high heat for 5 minutes.

If you like your vegetables semi-raw, serve at once, if not, turn down heat, cover and steam gently over a low heat for another 3–5 minutes. Before serving, add the seeds and toss again gently. Serve as soon as possible after cooking as a light lunch or with chops or poached fish as a main dish.

Hot runner beans with sesame (serves 2–3)
1 tbsp sesame seeds   *1 tbsp olive oil*
8 oz/225 g runner beans

Dry-roast the sesame seeds by stirring them in a heavy-based pan over a high heat for a few minutes, or until they begin to go brown. Set aside. Cook the runner beans in water until just tender. Drain the beans and reserve the juice for another recipe. Add a tablespoon of olive oil and the seeds and mix well. Serve at once.

Variation
Use thinly sliced Brussels sprouts, thick chunks of courgette, or florets of broccoli or cauliflower in place of the beans.

DESSERTS

Apple purée (serves 4)
1 lb/450 g apples
water (about ½ pt/250 ml)

Cut out any bad flesh from the apples and peel and core them. Cover the bottom of a large saucepan with water. Add the apples. Bring to boil and simmer covered until the apples are soft. Leave to cool, then sieve or liquidise. Keep in the fridge, or freeze in small plastic pots. This makes a thick puree which can be thinned out with apple juice to suit your recipe.

Variations
1. Sweeten with honey.
   2. Add raisins and/or ground mixed nuts and a little mixed spice.
   3. Add a crumble topping and bake.

NOTE: This is a good way to use up windfalls or bruised apples, or those that have been lingering in the fruit bowl too long.

Crumble topping

NOTE: This is a useful topping for fruit crumbles, fruit salads, fruit purées, etc. Make the dry mixture and keep in the fridge or freezer.

Dry mixture
Choose one of these:
  stale rye bread slices
  crumbled rye crispbreads
One of these:
  rolled oats
  barley flakes
  rye flakes
  millet flakes
  soya flakes
  wheat-free, sugar-free breakfast cereals
One of these:
  rice flour
  ground rice

Crush selected ingredients into a powder with a rolling pin in a plastic bag, or grind in a food processor or blender.

Ways to use the dry mixture
Hot topping
Take as much as you need and toss in olive oil or melted margarine and honey until the crumbs just stick together. Do not make the mixture too sticky. Spread over cooked fruit and bake in a moderate oven (180°C/230°F/gas mark 4) until brown.

Cold topping
Toss in oil or melted margarine (see above) and cook in a saucepan for a few minutes, turning continuously. Put into a dish and leave to cool. Sprinkle over fruit salad, sorbet or purée as required. Spare mixture can be kept fresh in the fridge for 3–4 days.

Custard

2 tsps cornflour
a little water
1 pt/570 ml almond
  milk (see page p. 245)
  or soya milk

1 egg
1 tbsp honey (or 2 tsps
  fructose)
a few drops of vanilla
  essence

Make a paste with the cornflour and a little water in a
small bowl. Heat milk gently until nearly boiling. Add
cornflour mixture to the hot milk and stir vigorously
until the flour is cooked and the mixture is slightly thickened. Remove from heat. Add beaten egg and stir well.
Place over a low heat and cook gently, stirring constantly
with a wooden spoon until smooth and thick. Add honey
(or fructose) to taste and vanilla essence. Serve at
once.

Fresh fruit salad

Choose any *four* of the following:
  1 dessert apple, sliced
  2 thick slices of pineapple
  1 banana
  ½ lb/225 g cherries, stoned
  ½ lb/225 g grapes, stoned and halved
  ½ lb/225 g of any soft fruits, e.g. raspberries,
    strawberries
  2 kiwi fruit, peeled and sliced
  1 pear, peeled and sliced
  1 orange, peeled, segmented and roughly chopped
  ½ a grapefruit, peeled, segmented and roughly
    chopped
  2 satsumas, peeled and segmented
juice of 1 lemon
1 tbsp clear honey
about ½ pt/275 ml orange or pineapple juice

Select and prepare fruit, and place in large bowl. Toss in
enough lemon juice to coat the fruit. Mix clear honey
with some of the orange or pineapple juice. Pour mixture

279

over the fruit. Add more juice to almost cover the fruit. Mix well and chill. Serve within 2 hours of preparation.

Variation
For a special occasion, add 2 tablespoonfuls of Cointreau or kirsch.

Fruit flan (to fill a 10–12 inch flan dish)
1 lb/450 g sweet non-wheat
  pastry (see page 247)
at least 1 lb/450 g fresh
  strawberries or
  raspberries (or 2 cans
  of apricots or peaches
  in fruit juice, drained)

Arrowroot glaze
¼ pt/150 ml lemon juice   *1 tsp clear honey*
1 tsp arrowroot

To make non-wheat pastry base: Preheat oven to 200°C/400°F/gas Mark 6. Roll out pastry gently and evenly and use to line a 10–12-inch/30 cm oven-proof flan dish. Bake blind for about 20 minutes or until lightly browned. Allow to cool.

If using canned fruit, drain well and reserve juice for arrowroot glaze. If using fresh fruit, halve any very large strawberries. When flan case is cool, pile or arrange the fruit attractively on the pastry base. Cover with a generous quantity of arrowroot glaze.

To make arrowroot glaze: Measure ¼ pt/150 ml juice reserved from canned fruit or lemon juice. Blend arrowroot with the juice and pour into a saucepan. Bring to the boil, stirring constantly, until the glaze is clear. Remove from heat and leave to cool a little before pouring over fruit.

Pineapple sorbet (serves 4)

1 large ripe pineapple, peeled and roughly chopped	3 tbsps clear honey 1 pt/570 ml water 1 egg white

Heat water and honey together gently and then boil for 2 minutes. Liquidise whole of pineapple flesh in this syrup. Put into shallow container and freeze until solid around the edges. (This should take about 30 minutes in the fast-freeze compartment of a deep freeze, but will take longer on the open shelves.)

Whisk egg white until stiff. Tip semi-solid pineapple mixture into a bowl and, using a wooden spoon, mix gently but thoroughly with the egg white. Place mixture in a plastic container, cover with a lid, cling film or aluminium foil and freeze until solid (approximately 2 hours). Remove from freezer and allow the sorbet to thaw for a few minutes before serving.

For an impressive dessert, scoop out flesh from the pineapple leaving shell intact. Fill shell with the sorbet and decorate with strawberries or raspberries. (Taken from Rose Elliot, *The Complete Vegetarian Cookbook*.)

NOTE: A soft, rather mushy sorbet can be made using this recipe in an ice-cream maker.

Quick fruit salad (serves 4–6)

1 banana, sliced 4 oz/100 g grapes, halved and seeded 1 dessert apple, sliced 14 oz/400 g tin of pineapple in fruit juice	14 oz/400 g tin of apricots in fruit juice juice of one lemon

Chop or slice fresh fruit. Toss in lemon juice to prevent browning. Open cans of tinned fruit and tip into a bowl with their juice. Add the lemon juice and fresh fruit and mix well. Serve as soon as possible.

Rhubarb and rice layer (serves 4)

1 lb/450 g rhubarb,
  chopped
4 tbsps date purée (see
  page 248)
1 tbsp grated orange rind
  (made from unwaxed
  organic orange if
  possible)

2 tbsps honey
at least 8 oz/225 g
  left-over cooked brown
  rice

Cut rhubarb into small pieces. Cook until tender and strain, reserving juice. Add the date purée and the rest of the orange juice to the cooked rhubarb and mix well. Check sweetness and adjust by adding honey.

Put about one-third of the cooked rice into the bottom of a baking dish and pour over half of the rhubarb mixture, add another third of the rice and pour over the rest of the rhubarb mixture. Top with remaining rice. Drizzle clear honey over the topping and bake at 200°C/400°F/gas mark 6 for about 25 minutes.

SWEET TREATS

Date and apricot loaf
(This is a filling, high-fibre cake, good for picnics or packed lunches.)

3 oz/75 g dried dates
4 oz/100 g dried apricots
½ pt/275 ml apple juice
2 oz/50 g whole almonds
4 oz/100 g sultanas

4 oz/100 g rice flour
1 tsp baking powder
¼ tsp mixed spice
1 oz/25 g oatbran
1 egg

Chop apricots and dates and soak overnight in apple juice. The next day, chop or roughly grind the almonds. Mix sultanas, flour, baking powder, spice and oatbran together in a large bowl. Add almonds, beaten eggs and apricot date mixture, and mix well. Put into a lined greased 1 lb/450 g loaf tin. Bake for about 1 hour at

180°C/350°F/ gas mark 4. The cake will be cooked when a skewer comes out clean. Leave until completely cold and serve in thick slices with vegan margarine. (Adapted from several similar recipes and tried out by a few of my trials candidates, to loud applause from their children!)

Fruit loaf (made without eggs)

4 oz/100 g raisins,
   cooked in a little water
4 oz/100 g rice flour
4 oz/100 g oatflakes
3 tbsps olive oil
pinch of salt

2 oz/50 g of desiccated
   coconut
2 oz/50 g chopped nuts
½ pt/275 ml of thick
   apple purée (see
   page 277)

Cook raisins in a little water and allow to cool. Mix flour, oatflakes, salt and oil. Add coconut and chopped nuts. Mix well. Add raisins and enough apple puree to make a soft dropping consistency. Spoon into a greased 1 lb/450 g loaf tin and bake for 1½ hours at 160°C/ 325°F/ gas mark 3, or until firm to the touch. Leave in the tin until quite cold before turning out. Use within a week.

Flapjacks

(This recipe was very popular among the trials candidates in 1988)

2 oz/50 g fruit sugar
2 tbsps maple syrup
4 oz/100 g vegan
   margarine

2 oz/50 g raisins
8 oz/225 g rolled oats

Heat sugar, syrup and margarine gently in a small saucepan. Add the oats and raisins and mix well together. Press into a shallow tin and bake at 180°C/350°F/gas mark 4, for 25 minutes. Allow to cool for 5 minutes before cutting into squares. Leave in tin until quite cold. (Gratefully received from one of my trials candidates who successfully adapted her favourite recipe.)

No-cook fruity nibbles (makes about 60 small sweets)

12 oz/350 g mixed dried
   fruits
4 oz/100 g mixed nuts
4 oz/100 g desiccated
   coconut
grated rind of carefully
   washed orange or
   lemon (unwaxed if
   possible)
a little orange juice

extra desiccated coconut
   for coating

Put dried fruits and nuts into a food processor until finely chopped. Then add coconut and grated rind and process again, adding enough orange juice to make a firm paste. Sprinkle a little desiccated coconut over the base of an 8 in/20 cm square tin, press fruit and nut mixture evenly over the base, then sprinkle with more coconut and press down well. Put a weight on top and place in fridge to firm up. Then slice into 1 in/2 cm squares. (Adapted from Rose Elliot, *The Complete Vegetarian Cookbook*.)

CHRISTMAS RECIPES

Christmas cake

date purée made from
   6 oz/175 g dried dates,
   cooked
4 oz/100 g dried apricots,
   soaked overnight,
   drained and chopped
4 oz/100 g prunes,
   soaked overnight,
   drained, stoned and
   chopped
6 oz/175 g vegan
   margarine

5 eggs, beaten
3 oz/75 g cornflour
3 oz/75 g rice flour
1 tsp mixed spice
3 oz/75 g almonds
rind and juice of 1 lemon
   (preferably unwaxed)
rind and juice of 1 orange
   (preferably unwaxed)
8 oz/225 g currants
6 oz/175 g raisins
6 oz/175 g sultanas

2 oz/50 g flaked almonds
2 tbsps white wine or
  brandy to pour
  over cooked cake.

The night before, prepare date purée, soak the prunes and apricots, drain them and chop them, reserving the juice to use as a drink mixed with orange juice.

The next day, pre-heat the oven to 150°C/300°F/gas mark 2. Grease and line a 9-inch/23 cm cake tin with grease-proof paper. Wrap brown paper around the outside of the tin and secure with string.

Beat date purée and margarine until creamy. Add the beaten eggs. Add the flour and spices and beat well. Add the rest of the ingredients, but not the brandy. Put mixture into a loaf tin and bake for 4–5 hours. Test to see if it is cooked by pushing a skewer into the centre. The cake will be cooked if it comes out cleanly.

Allow to cool on a wire rack. When cool, remove paper and turn cake out of the tin. When completely cold, turn the cake over and pour white wine or brandy over the base and allow to soak in. Wrap well in grease-proof paper and keep in an airtight tin until Christmas.

Mincemeat

4 oz/100 g currants
4 oz/100 g raisins
4 oz/100 g sultanas
2 oz/50 g cooking dates,
  finely chopped
4 oz/100 g grated apple
  or pear
grated rind of ½ a lemon
grated rind of ½ an
  orange
2 oz/50 g flaked almonds

1 ripe banana, mashed
6–8 oz/175–225 g of beef
  suet, or vegetable
  shortening, or 2–3
  tbsps of olive oil
¼ tsp each of ground
  ginger, grated nutmeg
  and mixed spice
4 tbsps of cider, apricot
  brandy or kirsch

Mix all ingredients thoroughly and place in screwtop jars. Use within two weeks.

The Calci-Counter

When you are shopping or planning your meals, buy as many foods as you can from the calcium-rich groups and fewer of the foods lower in calcium. Try to buy at least a few from the top four calcium groups every week, and try not to rely on foods that contain less than 20 mg calcium for each 100 g. Notice how many of your favourite food ingredients are in group C8! (*Source*: R.A. McCance and E.M. Widdowson, *The Composition of Foods* (HMSO, 1980)

CALCIUM FROM THE FOUR ZERO FOODS (GRAMS PER 100 G OF FOOD)

COWS' MILK

butter	15	dried milk	1020
Cheddar cheese	800	ice cream	140
cows', whole, raw	120	yoghurt	143
cream	79	(human milk)	(31)
curd/cottage cheese	60		

WHEAT

wheatbran	110	white flour,	
wheatgerm	17	unfortified	15
wholemeal flour	35		

BEET AND CANE SUGAR

demerara cane sugar	53	granulated	2
golden syrup	26	treacle	500

THE NIGHTSHADE FAMILY

aubergines, raw	10	potato chips	11
capsicum peppers	9	tomatoes	13
potatoes	8		

CALCIUM FROM SOME OF THE 200 FOODS

C1 (more than 500 mg per 100 g)

Fish

sardines, canned	550	whitebait, fried	860
sprats, fried	710		

Seeds

caraway seeds	689	(1 tsp 34)
cinnamon powder	1228	(1 tsp 61)
coriander seeds	709	(1 tsp 35)
dill seeds	1516	(1 tsp 76)
fennel seeds	1196	(1 tsp 60)
sesame seeds	783	(1 tsp 7)

Vegetables

spinach, boiled	600

C2 (300–500 mg per 100 g)

Fish

pilchards, canned	330	shrimps, boiled	320

Seeds

mustard powder	330

Beans and pulses
tofu   507

Vegetables
parsley   330   vine leaves   391

C3 (150–300 mg per 100 g)

Fish
anchovies   299   oysters   190
fish paste   280   prawns, boiled   150
mussels, boiled   220

Meat
tripe   150

Milk
sheep's   183

Nuts and seeds
almonds   250   nutmeg   184
brazils   180

Beans and pulses
red kidney beans   140   soya flour   210
soya beans   257

Vegetables
Chinese leaves   150   kale   212
dandelion leaves   158   watercress   220

Fruit
figs dried, raw   280   figs dried, stewed 160

C4 (101–150 mg per 100 g)

Fish
cockles, boiled   130   haddock, fried   110
crab, canned   120   scallops   120

| shrimps, canned | 110 | winkles, boiled | 140 |
| shrimps, frozen | 128 | | |

Meat
| pig's trotters | 129 |

Eggs
| chicken egg, yolk | 140 |

Nuts
| pistachio nuts | 140 |

Seeds
| sesame seeds | 131 |

Beans and pulses
| black-eyed peas | 110 | mung beans | 100 |
| cocoa powder | 130 | | |

Vegetables
broccoli tops	100	horseradish, raw	120
chives	129	spinach, canned	118
fennel leaves	109	spring onions	140

Fruit
| lemons, whole | 110 | rhubarb, raw | 100 |

Milk
| goats' | 130 |

C5 (51–100 mg per 100 g)

Fish
haddock, smoked	57	prawn, fresh	79
kipper, baked	65	salmon, canned	93
lemon sole, fried	95	sardines, cooked	85
lobster, boiled	62	skate, fried	50
mussels	88	whelks	54
plaice, fried	93		

Meat
meat paste   86

Eggs

chicken's, whole	52	duck's, whole	64

Nuts

peanuts	61	macadamia nuts	51
pecan	73	walnuts	61

Beans and pulses

chickpeas, cooked	67	soy sauce	65
haricot beans	65	soya milk	60

Vegetables

broccoli tops	76	red cabbage	53
celery, cooked	52	salsify	60
celery, raw	52	savoy cabbage	53
kohlrabi	68	spinach, raw	93
leeks, boiled	61	spring greens	86
mustard and cress	66	turnip tops	98
olives, whole	61	turnips, boiled	55
onions, fried	61		

Fruit

apricots, dried	92	dates, dried	68
blackberries, raw	63	raisins	61
blackberries, stewed	54	raspberries	61
blackcurrants, raw	60	rhubarb, stewed	84
blackcurrants, stewed	51	sultanas	52
currants	95		

Grains

millet flour	40	oats	80
oatcakes	54	pot barley	50
oatmeal	55	rye crispbread	50

Other foods

Marmite	95	yeast, dried	80

C6 (26–50 mg per 100 g)

Fish

cod, poached	29	salmon, steamed	29
crab, boiled	29	skate, fresh	40
herring, fried	39	sprats, fresh	39
herring, grilled	33	trout, steamed	36
mackerel, fried	28	tuna, fresh	40
plaice, steamed	38	whiting, fresh	42
rock salmon	39		

Meat

Bovril	40	pigeon	16
canned meats	9–32	sweetbreads	34
grouse	30	tongue	32
partridge	41	venison	29
pheasant	49		

Nuts

cashews	38	hazelnuts	44
chestnuts	46	peanut butter	37
coconut milk	29		

Vegetables

artichokes, globe	40	gooseberries, raw	28
asparagus	26	Jerusalem artichokes	30
beetroot, boiled	30	kale, boiled	48
Brussels sprouts	25	onions, raw	43
cabbage, white, raw	44	parsnips, boiled	36
carrot juice	27	peas, frozen, boiled	31
carrots, boiled	48	radishes	44
carrots, canned	27	runner beans	27
celeriac	47	seaweed (laverbread)	20
courgettes	30	shallots	26
endive	44	spring cabbage	30
French beans	39	swedes, boiled	42
garlic	38	winter cabbage	38

Fruit

apricots, stewed	34	prunes, raw	38
figs, fresh	34	pumpkin	39
loganberries, stewed	32	raspberries	41
mulberries	36	redcurrants, raw	36
oranges	41	tangerines	42
peaches, dried	36		

Grains

rye flour	32

C7 (11–25 mg per 100 g)

Fish

cod, steamed	15	haddock, fresh	18
cod's roe, fried	17	halibut, steamed	13
eel	21	salmon, smoked	19

Meat

bacon	7–16	hare/rabbit	11–21
brains	11–16	kidney	8–16
chicken	11	liver	6–15
duck	12	oxtail	14

Nuts

coconut, desiccated	22	coconut, fresh	13

Beans and pulses

butter beans	19	peas, dried, boiled	24
lentils, cooked	13		

Vegetables

avocado	15	cucumber	23
beansprouts	19	gherkin	25
broad beans	21	horseradish, raw	20
cauliflower, boiled	18	lettuce	23
chicory, raw	8	marrow, boiled	14

mushrooms, boiled	24	runner beans	22
peas, canned	24	sweet potatoes	21
peas, fresh, boiled	13	waterchestnuts	18

Fruit

apricots, raw	17	honeydew melon	14
cantaloupe melon	19	limes	13
cherries, raw	16	mandarins, canned	18
cherries, stewed	18	peaches, dried, stewed	13
cranberries	15	pineapple	12
damsons, raw	24	plums, raw	11–14
damsons, stewed	20	plums, stewed	18
grapefruit	17	pomegranates	13
grapes, white	19	quinces	14
greengages, raw	17	strawberries	22

Grains

buckwheat	21	rice flakes	20
cornflour	15	rice, ground	24
rice, brown	23	rye bread	23

Other

yeast, fresh	25

C8 (10 mg or less per 100 g)

Fish

halibut	10

Meat

chicken	10	pork	8
goose	10	turkey	9
lamb/mutton	7	heart	5–10

Vegetables

mushrooms, raw	3	sweetcorn, boiled	4

Fruits

apple juice	8	mangoes, canned	10
apples, raw	3–4	nectarines	4
bananas	7	peaches, raw	5
bilberries	10	pears, raw	6
grapes, black	4	watermelon	4
lemon juice	8	yam	10
lychees, raw	8		

Grains and starch foods

arrowroot	7	porridge	6
boiled white rice	1	rice flour	7
pearl barley	10	sago	10
polished rice	4	tapioca	8

Eggs

chicken's, raw white	5

Sweeteners

honey	5

Useful Books

Food
Chaitow, Leon *Stone Age Diet* (Optima books, 1987).
Everkus, Carol, *et al.*, *The Great British Diet* (Century, 1985).
Griggs, Barbara, *The Food Factor* (Penguin, 1988).
Hetzel, Basil, and McMichael, Tony, *The LS factor* (Penguin (Australia), 1987).
Mervyn, Leonard, *Calcium and Osteoporosis* (Thorsons, 1988).
Mindell, Earl, *The Vitamin Bible* (Arlington Books, 1987).
Williams, Xandria, *What's in My Food?* (Prism Press, Australia, 1988).

Slimming
Kenton, Leslie, *The Biogenic Diet* (Arrow, 1986).
Paterson, Barbara, *The A for Allergy Diet Book* (Corgi, 1986).

Addiction
Mackarness, Richard, *A Little of What You Fancy* (Fontana, 1985).

Food intolerance and allergies
Brostoff, John, *Food Allergy and Intolerance* (Bloomsbury, 1989).

Buist, Robert, *Food Intolerance and How to Cope with It* (Collins, Australia, 1984).

Davies, Stephen, and Stewart, Alan, *Nutritional Medicine* (Pan, 1987).

Mackarness, Richard, *Not All in the Mind* (Pan, 1976).

Paterson, Barbara, *The Allergy Connection* (Thorsons, 1984).

Randolph, Theron, and Moss, Ralph, *Allergies: Your Hidden Enemy* (Thorsons, 1984).

Seely, Stephen, *et al.*, *Diet-Related Diseases* (Croom Helm, 1985).

Premenstrual tension
Dalton, Katharine, *Once a Month* (Fontana, 1987).

Eating
Bennet, Gerald, *Eating Matters* (Heinemann Kingswood, 1988).

Colbin, Annemarie, *Food and Healing* (Ballantine Books, New York, 1986).

Maisner, Pauline, *The Food Trap* (Unwin Paperbacks, 1986).

Feeding the family: children
Lobstein, Tim, *Children's Food* (Unwin Paperbacks, 1988).

Minchin, Maureen, *Food for Thought* (Oxford University Press, 1984).

Useful Addresses

Using soya products
For information, send SAE to:
  Soya Milk Information Bureau
  The Chestnuts
  Fosse Way
  Moreton Morrell
  Warks CV35 9DE

Foresight: The Association for Pre-conceptual Care
For the address of your nearest Foresight clinic, send SAE to:
  The Secretary
  Foresight
  The Old Vicarage
  Church Lane
  Witley
  Surrey GU8 5PN
(Useful booklet available: *Guidelines for Future Parents*.)

Living without milk
For booklist and advice about living without milk, send SAE to:
  The Vegan Society
  33–35 George St
  Oxford OX1 2AY

Hyperactive children

For information about local support groups, send SAE to:

    The Hyperactive Children's Support Group
    71 Whyke Lane
    Chichester
    West Sussex PO19 2LD

Foods by mail order

For mailing list and information, send SAE to:

    Foodwatch International
    Butts Pond Industrial Estate
    Sturminster Newton
    Dorset DT10 1AZ

References

Chapter 1   Four Zero Foods

1. Health Education Council, *Proposals for Nutritional Guidelines for Health Education in Britain* (HMSO, 1983).

2. Mervyn, Leonard, *Calcium and Osteoporosis* (Thorsons, 1988) p. 42 (MAFF statistics).

3. Brostoff, John, *Food Allergy and Intolerance* (Bloomsbury, 1989), p. 266.

4. Seely, Stephen, *et al.*, *Diet-related Diseases* (Croom Helm, 1985), p. 144.

5. Williams, Xandria, *What's in My Food?* (Prism Press, 1988), p. 179.

6. Mervyn, op. cit., pp. 70–2.

7. ibid., p. 40.

8. Seely *et al.*, op. cit., p. 52.

9. ibid., p. 52.

Chapter 2   You and Your Health

1. Seely, Stephen, *et al.*, *Diet-related Diseases* (Croom Helm, 1985), pp. 239–41.

Chapter 3   You and Your Food

1. BUPA Medical Centre leaflet, *The Facts about Drinking and How to Control It*.

2. Hanssen, Maurice, *E for Additives* (Thornsons, 1986).

3. Griggs, Barbara, *The Food Factor*, ch. 9. Gives details of the Bircher-Benner diet, based on raw food.

Chapter 10   Tackling Other Addictions

1. Brostoff, John, *Food Allergy and Intolerance* (Bloomsbury, 1989), p. 159.

2. Davies, Stephen and Stewart, Alan, *Nutritional Medicine* (Pan, 1987), p. 137

3. Ibid., p. 349.

Starting a Winners' Group

Once you have seen the benefits of following the Food Addict's Diet, you may feel that you want to spread the message a little further. One way to do this is to start a local Winners' Group.

WHAT IS A WINNERS' GROUP?

Coping with food addiction can be a lonely, rather confusing business for some people. In particular, those with eating disorders or a chronic weight problem need a great deal of support and advice to follow the diet consistently for long enough to solve their particular problem.

Winners' Groups are small self-help groups of between four and twelve people, set up by some of those who have completed the four zero experiment and are familiar with the diet (see below).

Meetings will be arranged on a six-week rolling programme, and you will be invited to join in week 1 or 2. Although this may mean a considerable delay before you can join, the advantage is that most of the group members will be at about the same stage of the diet. In weeks 1 and 2 group members will be either beginning the diet or making a fresh start after a break with the restart plan, and the other members who are well established on the Food Addict's Diet can provide valuable support and advice to the others.

Our experiences on the pilot Winners' Group have shown clearly that the initial six meetings are crucial to the success of the diet, after which only occasional attendance is needed. However, for members with greater problems, several months of support may be required before their addictions are firmly under their control.

There is a registration fee which makes you a member of the group for one year, and which will be handed over at your first group meeting. (The group leader will advise you about this when you first make contact with him/her.) Apart from that, all you will have to pay is a small donation directly to the group leader towards the costs of any light refreshments provided.

FINDING A WINNERS' GROUP IN YOUR AREA

If there is no Winners' Group in your area, I suggest that you follow the diet with a friend and support one another. If you keep a close eye on the local press and ask around among your associates, you may eventually hear of a local group starting up.

In the early days, while the number of groups is very small, you may have difficulty finding one, and in that case the only way to join a group will be to start one.

BECOMING A GROUP LEADER

If you decide that you would like to set up a Winners' Group, send for an information pack to:

'Winners'
PO Box no. 396
St Albans
Herts AL3 6NE

(Information packs can only be sent to those who enclose a stamped, self-addressed A4 envelope.)

Once you know exactly what will be involved, and if you still want to apply to be a group leader, you will be asked to fill in another form, provided with the information pack, giving a little more information about yourself. You then send it back to us.

Those who wish to start a group must be able to show that they are totally familiar with the details of each chapter of this book. Initially they will be asked to help one other person through the four zero experiment, including the rest test and the restart plan, and send in a weekly progress report for the first six weeks.

No special qualifications are needed: just a sympathetic personality, one spare evening a week, and available space for an average of eight group members to meet, in your home or elsewhere. Once we are satisfied that you have the necessary skills, then you will be allocated a group number and you are free to recruit up to a maximum of twelve members either by personal contact or a local advertisement. Regular, on-going support and advice will be available to Winners' Group leaders on a pre-arranged basis.

Being a group leader is voluntary and unpaid, although for some highly experienced group leaders there may be the possibility of promotion to a part-time paid post as local or district adviser as the national network expands.

GOING TO YOUR FIRST MEETING

When you have found a local group, and have been given a date to go to your first meeting, take with you the form at the back of the book (not a photocopy) to prove that you are a *bona fide* purchaser of this book: you cannot join without it.

Index

WINNERS REGISTRATION FORM

I would like to apply to join your Winners' Group.

NAME . . . .
ADDRESS . . . .
. . . .
. . . .
. . . .

TELEPHONE NUMBER . . . .

My special interest(s) in the diet is (tick):
Slimming
Other addictions
Food intolerance
Eating disorder
Premenstrual tension
Children's health
Partner's health
Other . . . .

I agree to pay the current registration fee.
SIGNED . . . .
DATED . . . .